Using Natural Remedies Safely in Pregnancy and Childbirth

by the same author

Aromatherapy in Midwifery Practice
ISBN 978 1 84819 288 1
eISBN 978 0 85701 235 7

Complementary Therapies in Maternity Care
An Evidence-Based Approach
ISBN 978 1 84819 328 4
eISBN 978 0 85701 284 5

The Business of Maternity Care
A Guide for Midwives and Doulas Setting Up in Private Practice
ISBN 978 1 84819 386 4
eISBN 978 0 85701 385 9

of related interest

Supporting Survivors of Sexual Abuse Through Pregnancy and Childbirth
A Guide for Midwives, Doulas and Other Healthcare Professionals
Kicki Hansard
Forewords by Penny Simkin and Phyllis Klaus
ISBN 978 1 84819 424 3
eISBN 978 0 85701 377 4

Using Natural Remedies Safely in Pregnancy and Childbirth

A REFERENCE GUIDE FOR MATERNITY AND HEALTHCARE PROFESSIONALS

Denise Tiran

FOREWORD BY PAM CONRAD

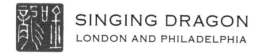

SINGING DRAGON
LONDON AND PHILADELPHIA

Disclaimer: The use of complementary therapy practice within maternity care is constantly evolving in response to the needs of women, their families and caregivers, research evidence and service demands and in relation to developments in obstetrics. It is the responsibility of the midwife, doula, complementary therapist or other professional practitioner to remain updated, to engage in evidence-based practice and to work within the parameters of her/his own clinical practice. The author and publisher are not responsible for any harm or damage to a person, no matter how caused, as a result of information shared in this book.

First published in Great Britain in 2021 by Singing Dragon,
an imprint of Jessica Kingsley Publishers
An Hachette Company

1

The information contained in this book is not intended to replace the services of trained medical professionals or to be a substitute for medical advice. The complementary therapy described in this book may not be suitable for everyone to follow. You are advised to consult a doctor before embarking on any complementary therapy programme and on any matters relating to your health, and in particular on any matters that may require diagnosis or medical attention.

A CIP catalogue record for this title is available from the British Library and the Library of Congress

ISBN 978 1 78775 252 8
eISBN 978 1 78775 253 5

Printed and bound in Great Britain by Clays Ltd

Jessica Kingsley Publishers' policy is to use papers that are natural, renewable and recyclable products and made from wood grown in sustainable forests. The logging and manufacturing processes are expected to conform to the environmental regulations of the country of origin.

Jessica Kingsley Publishers
Carmelite House
50 Victoria Embankment
London EC4Y 0DZ

www.singingdragon.com

As always, this book is dedicated to my wonderful son, Adam, still living and working in the music industry in our beloved South Africa. As I complete the manuscript for this book, the 2020 coronavirus pandemic rages and the whole world is in lockdown – come home safely soon. I miss you.

Contents

Foreword

The hunger for natural therapies and self-care remedies has exploded globally amongst women, and particularly those on the significant journey towards motherhood: the pregnant woman. Unfounded claims for enhancing fetal development and easing the childbirth experience are promoted by well-intentioned, albeit under-educated individuals, potentially leading to unnecessary risk factors at a vulnerable time. Capitalizing on this trend, herbal and aromatherapy companies market heavily to this segment of the population often without adequate knowledge to safely guide them. This book, written by the foremost authority on the safe use of natural remedies during the pregnancy–childbirth–postnatal period, Denise Tiran, could not be more timely.

Since the late 1980s, Denise Tiran, a registered midwife, practitioner and university educator, has qualified in aromatherapy, herbal medicine, homeopathy, reflex zone therapy, Bach Flower Remedies and a myriad of midwifery techniques, all to improve the experience of pregnancy and childbirth for thousands of women. A pioneer and leading expert in the field, she has written over 15 books and multiple papers for midwifery and complementary or alternative medicine (CAM) practice, and again this book is one of her finest, a true gem.

As I read through the book whilst continuing to learn from Denise, I am reminded of my clinical aromatherapy internship as a nurse and newly qualified aromatherapist nearly 20 years ago with her at Queen Mary's Hospital, London. Transferred to England because of my husband's job, having just devoured her unrivalled *Aromatherapy for Pregnancy and Childbirth* book, the fortunate opportunity to observe and practise alongside her for a year bridged the gap of understanding integrative medicine and how to specifically weave these therapies into traditional nursing and midwifery care. Twenty years later, thousands of US women have benefited from this unique opportunity of learning that now has been taught to nurses, midwives and doulas, and with this book it can spread even further.

The wealth of information in this book provides midwives, nurses and maternity healthcare professionals with timely and much needed specific herbal, homeopathic and select essential oil information to initiate dialogue with our patients and guide the assessment of the appropriateness for natural remedies with each unique and often changing clinical scenario. Her prenatal CAM clinic at Queen Mary's Hospital, London, where I interned, treated a vast array of multicultural women, and her knowledge of and respect for their traditional medicine systems encouraged open dialogue, education and safer outcomes, and are thoughtfully included in this book.

Herbal medicine, homeopathy and aromatherapy all fall under the category of "natural medicines" and the umbrella of CAM. In the USA, homeopathy and herbal medicine lack standardized education or a credentialing body for professional practice, so it is not uncommon to hear a homeopathic or herbal remedy referred to as if they were one and the same. This book clarifies the unique and most important differences to expertly guide the individual or practitioner. The majority of the time, individuals self-treat from a health food shop without professional guidance. This is of particular concern during pregnancy, childbirth and lactation when the risk factors are greater.

Women seeking natural alternatives often arrive at the labour suite with bags of various remedies unknown to their healthcare team or clearly understood by them. This book does a marvellous job of differentiating the potency and risk factors between a herb, homeopathic, flower remedy or essential oil, even those possessing the same name (i.e. chamomile, ginger, peppermint) but with very different potency, safety and risk factors.

Aromatherapy, the most popular of the natural remedies, is highlighted for its wide range of uses in pregnancy, childbirth and postnatally with the necessary cautions for use. With often enthusiastic, albeit under-educated, essential oil sales and recommendations, particularly during pregnancy, this book will serve as a valuable tool for childbirth education.

This well-researched book provides in-depth information on multiple natural remedies that midwives, nurses, doulas, physicians and other health professionals can use clinically to advise, educate and inform the prenatal-postnatal women in their care, focusing on safety in their application.

The alphabetical listing of 220 remedies, with their common uses, precautions, potential interactions and contraindications for use specifically during the pregnancy, childbirth and postnatal period, make this a very valuable and practical book.

As I reflect on the wisdom and inspiration of Maya Angelou as it relates to this book, "Do the best you can until you know better, then when you know better, do better", I'm honoured to highly recommend this book to enrich our knowledge of natural therapies and, by doing so, we can encourage and educate the women in our care, as we now know a better way!

Pam Conrad PGd, BSN, RN, CCAP
Practitioner, educator, researcher, author
Indianapolis, Indiana, USA

Acknowledgements

I would like to thank everyone at Jessica Kingsley Publishers (JKP) for giving me the opportunity to write this latest book, particularly my editor, Sarah Hamlin, and her editorial assistant, Maddy Budd. I would also like to express my gratitude and good wishes to Claire Wilson, Editorial Director at JKP, with whom I have worked for many years and who saw the original proposal for this latest book. Thanks to all the midwives who have undertaken many of the complementary therapy courses provided by my company, Expectancy, for their kind and helpful suggestions for the book. It has been fascinating discussing natural remedies with colleagues during our study days and considering some of the issues for maternity professionals when working with women who use natural remedies or complementary therapies. In particular, I would like to thank my tutorial team at Expectancy, especially Amanda Redford and Laura Wallbank, for critically reviewing the manuscript and for their enormous support. Thank you also to my best friend, Alina, who has kept me sane, giving me a bed in Scotland with space to get away from my London office to continue writing, as well as the occasional medicinal gin and tonic!

How to Use this Book

This book is intended as a reference text for midwives, doctors, health visitors, doulas, maternity support workers, complementary therapists, pharmacists and other healthcare practitioners who have professional contact with pregnant women. Health professionals may be asked by women for information and advice on the safety of herbal and homeopathic medicines, aromatherapy essential oils and on the traditional plant, mineral and animal-based remedies used by women from different cultures. Maternity care providers may also elicit women's use of various remedies whilst caring for them and be unsure about the safety or appropriateness of the remedies at different times during pregnancy, labour or the postnatal period. Complementary practitioners from all disciplines may come into contact with pregnant clients who ask them about common remedies used in pregnancy, whilst pharmacists and salespersons in health stores may encounter pregnant customers who question them about natural remedies. Also, midwives and doulas may integrate various natural remedies into their care of women, especially aromatherapy and advice on herbs and homeopathy.

The emphasis in this book is on the *safety* of natural remedies in pregnancy, labour and postnatally, rather than on how to use them. It is often difficult to access information about safety. In this book I have used my extensive investigation of the safety of natural remedies and applied generic principles to the childbearing year – the preconception, antenatal, intrapartum and postnatal periods.

Chapter 1, the introductory chapter, provides an overview of the different systems of natural remedies, including their mechanisms of action and general indications, contraindications and precautions. Chapter 2 focuses on the use of natural remedies specifically in pregnancy and childbirth. In Chapter 3 I have debated the issue of risk and considered how health professionals, both conventional and complementary, can contribute to ensuring the safety of expectant, labouring and newly birthed mothers when they choose to use natural remedies. I have debated the issue of risk and considered how health professionals, both conventional and complementary, can contribute to ensuring the safety of expectant, labouring and newly birthed mothers when they choose to use natural remedies. A thorough investigation into the potential adverse effects, possible toxicity and interactions with other chemical substances makes for sobering reading but is intended to alert professionals to the pertinent advice that women may need in respect of natural remedies. The clear message is that "natural" does not necessarily mean "safe", especially in pregnancy. Guidelines for the safe use of natural remedies in pregnancy follow in Chapter 4, and the short answer to any doubts about safety is to avoid using them, at least until more specialist information can be obtained.

There follows an alphabetical listing of 220 natural remedies, for quick reference in clinical practice. These include primarily herbal and some homeopathic remedies, essential oils, mineral substances and a few remedies sourced from animals, particularly those used in traditional medicine in developing countries. There are many hundreds of remedies that could have been included, but I have explored a small selection of commonly used remedies, primarily in the developed world. The entries for each natural remedy have not been directly referenced in the text since the book is a "ready reference" for use in clinical practice. However, information has been sourced from a variety of academic and clinical resources, using the most up-to-date material available. References for Chapters 1–3 and a Glossary of Terms used in the alphabetical listings are given at the end of the book.

In the alphabetical listing of herbal and homeopathic remedies and mineral and animal products, each has several sections.

Herbal remedies (including essential oils and traditional remedies)

These entries identify the common or traditional uses, both obstetric-related and general, and their safety, specifically related to pregnancy, labour and breastfeeding. Most remedies are administered orally, but topical (dermal), inhalational or other methods of administration are also covered where appropriate. Some plant-based remedies are consumed within the diet and are generally considered safe enough in amounts commonly found in foods; safety information given within the profile applies primarily, but not solely, to therapeutic doses or incorrect use.

Contraindications and precautions are included, where necessary extrapolating data from the available information on general contraindications and applying them to pregnant and childbearing women. It must be emphasized that this book is intended mainly for maternity professionals, not for qualified medical herbalists and homeopaths, and there may appear to be some contradictions in these sections. An example of this would be raspberry leaf, in which the alphabetical entry advises avoiding self-administration until the third trimester (information which maternity carers should advise), whereas a medical herbalist may appropriately prescribe it under their own accountability for threatened first trimester miscarriage. Maternity professionals come into contact with many women who are self-prescribing and self-administering, and this book is intended to help maternity professionals err on the side of caution unless they are able to discuss individual cases with a qualified natural remedies (NR) practitioner.

The adverse effects section covers moderate and severe symptoms experienced both from therapeutic doses and from incorrect administration. The interactions section identifies possible pharmacological interactions with drugs and plant remedies, and occasionally with investigative medical tests. Interactions may be definitive or theoretical, usually occurring with therapeutic or recreational use, or from prolonged, excessive or inappropriate use, sometimes even in the amounts found in foods. These sections are included for all remedies, including those that are completely contraindicated, so that professionals can comprehensively advise women who reveal self-administration of herbs considered unsafe, or about which there is little evidence-based information. This may also be helpful for health professionals when apparently idiopathic untoward symptoms occur before, during or after childbirth.

Homeopathic remedies

In these listings, the main obstetric indications are identified, together with those coincidental conditions that women may experience during pregnancy, such as the common cold, accidental injury or ongoing pre-existing problems. There follows a key features section – these are the symptoms, manifestations and emotional aspects that would normally enable a homeopath to prescribe the most appropriate remedy. They are included here so that healthcare professionals working with pregnant women using homeopathy can assess whether or not they are using the correct remedy. For example, a midwife or doula may be caring for a woman self-administering a homeopathic remedy in labour, but since labour is a dynamic process, the indications for use of a specific remedy may change as the labour progresses. The initial remedy is therefore no longer valid, and continuing to self-administer it could lead either to new symptoms or could mask emerging clinical pathology. Two brief sections follow, on "better for" and "worse for", giving signs and symptoms that characterize whether the specific remedy is appropriate or not. Finally, the section on safety includes general information and any safety issues that have arisen or that apply to the specific remedy.

Mineral and animal products

A few remedies originating from mineral or animal products are included in the listings, using the same sub-headings as those for herbal remedies. Some of these remedies are traditional to specific cultures but the widespread use of the internet and the multicultural nature of populations in westernized countries may mean that healthcare professionals come into contact with women wishing to use them during pregnancy. Although there may be little or no research evidence on these remedies, safety information is extrapolated from what is known and the ways in which women use the remedies.

1

Introduction

Natural remedies (NRs) are derived from any naturally occurring substances and used for medicinal purposes. NRs comprise a significant part of the non-allopathic modalities that constitute "complementary and alternative medicine", although this broader term also encompasses manual, energetic and psychological therapies, such as massage, acupuncture and hypnotherapy, which are not dealt with in this book (for more on this, see Tiran 2018).

The most common forms of NRs are those used in medical herbalism, aromatherapy, energetic medicine modalities such as homeopathy and flower remedies, as well as various traditional medical systems from around the world. Some authorities would also include nutritional therapies, for example macrobiotics and vitamin and mineral supplements, in the general classification of "natural remedies". However, whilst some NRs can be used as culinary flavourings or may interact with certain foods, nutritional therapy is a completely different discipline and is not discussed in this book.

Most NRs are developed from plant materials, although mineral, bacterial and viral, lichens, algae and animal substances are also used, particularly in homeopathy and in traditional medicine systems. Plants have been part of folk medicine for centuries, especially for pregnancy and childbirth, and it has been claimed that there are around 350,000 plants worldwide, many with untapped medicinal potential (Heywood 2011). In the 17th century, the well-known herbalist, Nicholas Culpeper (1616–1652), was the first person to produce an English language herbal pharmacopoeia and, in 1651, a Directory for Midwives exploring popular remedies for reproduction, many of which are still in use today. Developments in medicine in the late 18th and early 19th centuries moved plant remedies on to a more professional setting that eventually evolved into the modern pharmaceutical sciences. From the 19th century, much of the empirical evidence was lost and science overtook the traditional ways of life. Since the late 20th century and into the 21st century, the medical and scientific fraternities have viewed NRs as part of complementary or alternative medicine (CAM).

Conversely, there has been a phenomenal resurgence in the public's use of NRs in the industrialized world in the past few decades as people seek a return to a more organic way of life, often rejecting the paternalistic bioscientific approach of allopathic medicine. Various contemporary surveys, systematic reviews and other studies show that the use of NRs ranges from around 35 per cent to 41 per cent of the general population in Europe, North America, Canada and the Middle East (Awad and Al-Shaye 2014; Rashrash, Schommer and Brown 2017; Welz, Emberger-Klein and Menrad 2018). Some reports claim that almost 70 per cent of Australians now embrace complementary medicine in general, but specific information on NR use, particularly in pregnancy, is less readily available (ATMS 2018).

Around the world the most commonly quoted indications for the use of NRs appear to be to promote and maintain general health and wellbeing, to treat minor illnesses and sometimes to attempt to resolve more serious conditions before, or instead of, seeking medical advice (Rahmawati and Bajorek 2017). However, definitive information is difficult to find because surveys use varying terms when posing questions to respondents. The term "natural remedies" may include solely herbal medicines (Zeni *et al.* 2017), or herbs and aromatherapy oils, or herbs and non-pharmacological modalities such as homeopathy (Awad and Al-Shaye 2014), or it may, somewhat erroneously, be interpreted as all elements of CAM including manual and manipulative therapies (Posadzki *et al.* 2013).

Similarly, the use of traditional medicines (TMs) continues in many parts of the world today. Russia has been described as having a "herbophilious" society, with around 58 per cent of the population preferring NRs to drugs, and most using medicinal plants as an integral part of their daily diet (Shikov *et al.* 2017). It is estimated that between 65 per cent and 85 per cent of rural populations in Africa, Asia and parts of South America use indigenous plants and other substances for medicinal purposes (Ekor 2013; WHO 2019; Zeni *et al.* 2017). Indeed, one survey claimed that almost 100 per cent of African women resort to plants for family medicines (S.M. Ahmed *et al.* 2018). In China and other Asian countries such as Japan, Korea and Vietnam, traditional Chinese medicine (TCM) and national and regional variations are often used concomitantly with conventional healthcare. Indeed, a huge credibility boost has recently been achieved through the acceptance of TM by the World Health Organization (WHO), despite critics claiming there is insufficient evidence to support its use (Hunt 2019).

Different systems of natural remedies
Herbal medicine
Herbal medicine, also known as botanical medicine or phytotherapy ("phyto" = plant), is the oldest therapeutic modality in the world, with archaeological evidence that it was used up to 60,000 years ago. It involves the preparation of fresh or dried plant materials to be administered in various formats. Kew Gardens in London estimates that, globally, over 28,000 plants are currently in use as medicines, although less than 20 per cent of these are included in formal medicinal publications such as pharmacopoeia (Royal Botanical Gardens, Kew 2017). This may be due to the lack of definitive research, scientific scepticism for some modalities that encompass plant remedies such as homeopathy, and the somewhat enigmatic medicinal use of many plants by culturally diverse groups in geographically disparate areas of the world as part of their traditional heritages (see "Homeopathy and energetic remedies" and "Traditional medicine systems", below).

Botanical medicines may be administered as liquid extracts or dried material, from the whole plant or from part of it, such as the leaf, fruit or root. They can be prepared by drying and formulating them into herbal teas or tisanes; essential oils are extracted, commonly by simple steam distillation or by more sophisticated processes. Other herbal products containing complex mixtures of compounds from the plant are processed into tablets, tinctures, creams, suppositories and pessaries. Plants contain numerous constituents which can have physiological effects, including astringent tannins, detoxifying, diuretics, hepatoprotective and hormone-regulating saponins, mucilages which soothe and protect the tissues, antioxidant flavonoids, hormone-like phytoestrogens, volatile (essential) oils and others. Efficacy, safety and purity of herbal remedies may depend on the climate and the soil in which the plants are grown, harvesting and production methods, national and international standardization and the presence or absence of contaminants such as pesticides, heavy metals or microbes.

All herbal medicines, including aromatherapy essential oils and herbal teas, have physiological effects. Irrespective of the method of administration, herbal medicines act systemically, being absorbed, distributed and metabolized, primarily via the liver; waste products are excreted via the kidneys, lungs and skin and to a lesser extent via the intestines (He, Chan and Zhou 2011). The amount of active chemical constituents in herbal remedies may depend on the format – for example, most herbal teas contain extremely diluted amounts of the active constituents compared to tablets or tinctures produced from the same plants in a formal therapeutic dose.

Medical herbalism in developed countries is based on fairly robust evidence of effectiveness and safety or on tried and trusted pharmacopoeia. Training, often at undergraduate or even Master's level, involves a comprehensive study of anatomy, physiopathology, chemistry, pharmacology, diagnostics, interactions between herbal and pharmaceutical medicines and, more recently, genetics and genomics. Medical herbalists are generally well respected, and although their practice is discrete from mainstream medicine, the scientific and medical communities are increasingly acknowledging the pharmacological nature of the remedies. Indeed, many conventional drugs have their origins in the isolation of chemical constituents from various plants, the first – morphine – being derived from the opium poppy over 200 years ago. Other drugs originating from plants include digitalis (digoxin) from the foxglove; the cancer drug, vincristine, from periwinkle; aspirin, the salicin content (a precursor to aspirin) being found in the bark of the willow tree; and the progesterone-only contraceptive Pill, derived from wild yam.

In the UK and most of Europe, herbal medicine has been regulated by the European Union (EU), which, in 2011, imposed a regulatory system across all member states. All manufactured herbal medicines, previously categorized as unlicensed, are required to have either traditional herbal registration or marketing authorization based on well-established use. Registered herbal medicines must meet specific standards of safety and quality and be accompanied by agreed indications from a minimum of 30 years of common usage; systematic patient safety information must be provided. Licensed herbal medicines have marketing authorization similar to the approval of conventional medicines, although the process is less rigorous than in the preparation of commercially produced pharmaceutical drugs. Nutritional supplements such as vitamins and minerals are not included in this system.

In the USA, herbal and other categories of natural medicine are regulated by the Food and Drug Administration (FDA), being categorized as nutritional supplements that do not require full licensing prior to sale. Some countries, such as Saudi Arabia, permit herbal remedies if they have a substantial period of traditional use – in this case, 50 years. Conversely, in Canada the Natural Health Products Directorate requires clear evidence of the composition and standardization of each product, methods of testing for contaminants, human tolerance limits and safety and effectiveness before approving a remedy for public sale. The Australian Register of Therapeutic Goods is responsible for approving for sale and use all natural medicines, medical devices and other products such as disinfectants. In other countries where recognized herbal remedies are used within the prevailing TM system, regulations may differ (see "Traditional medicine systems", below).

Aromatherapy essential oils

As part of herbal medicine, essential oils may be used in conjunction with other plant constituents. Medical herbalists can prescribe and administer essential oils as medicines for administration orally, via rectal suppositories or vaginal pessaries; many doctors in countries such as France prescribe essential oils as medicinal drugs. Essential oils have also previously been injected, both intravenously and subcutaneously, but this practice is now largely obsolete. However, these methods of administration must be carefully supervised and are not appropriate in pregnancy and childbirth unless under the guidance of a medical practitioner or an aromatologist who is qualified to administer essential oils.

In most countries, essential oils are more commonly used in isolation as part of the CAM modality of aromatherapy, in which highly concentrated volatile oils are extracted from various parts of different plants to be used topically and by inhalation, harnessing both the physiological effects of their chemical constituents and the psychological effects of their aromas.

Aromatherapy is extremely popular with the public, worth $1.8 billion in the USA in 2018 and expected to grow by 10 per cent by 2026 (Grand View Research 2019). Self-administration is the primary mode of use; in the UK, home use constitutes 45 per cent of the total aromatherapy market (Grand View Research 2019). The Asia Pacific region's demand for essential oils is set to rise exponentially, with a claim that, in India, this is due to the increasing number of industrial burns for which treatment with essential oils may be effective (Grand View Research 2019).

Unfortunately, the pleasant fragrances of essential oils and the popularity, in many countries, of administering them topically via massage means that aromatherapy has gained a reputation primarily as a relaxation therapy. This is not helped by the abundant use of essential oils in the beauty therapy and perfumery industries, and their ready availability for sale in shops and online, which detracts from the lay public's understanding of their pharmacological action, potential medicinal uses and risks.

Each essential oil contains several hundred different chemical constituents, with physiological and psychological effects arising from their pharmacological, that is, systemic, action. Many of the chemical constituents have proven anti-infective effects, some affect blood pressure, some are relaxing whilst others are stimulating, and some appear to have direct effects on blood cells (Assmann *et al.* 2018; Freeman *et al.* 2019; Kawai *et al.* 2020; Tariq *et al.* 2019). Once absorbed into the body, by whatever method of administration, the chemicals are metabolized via the liver; waste products are excreted via the renal, respiratory and integumentary systems (for more information on clinical aromatherapy in pregnancy, see Tiran 2016).

Regulatory systems of the aromatherapy profession vary around the world but tend to be via optional self-regulation rather than through statutory mechanisms. In many countries, the therapeutic use of essential oils falls under national cosmetics regulations, although in others they are regulated via drugs legislation. Training, standards and parameters of clinical practice vary between countries, as do the regulations for the sale of essential oils to the public. However, despite huge public use and a reasonable body of research evidence, aromatherapy is not considered as scientifically sound as some other therapies. This may be for several reasons. First, the association with the beauty and cosmetics industries seems to devalue aromatherapy as a clinical modality. Many studies explore the use of essential oils in vitro, such as laboratory testing of the anti-infective properties of specific oils (e.g. tea tree). There is limited clinical evidence, most of which investigates the concept of aromatherapy (e.g. "aromatherapy aids sleep" or "aromatherapy eases pain") in which the subjective client–therapist relationship or the placebo effect may also play a part. There are far fewer studies on the clinical use of specific essential oils for specific conditions. Research methodology varies and is sometimes poor, and there are wide disparities in the actual practice of aromatherapy between countries, which, in some cases, is questionable. Whilst some studies on effectiveness have been undertaken using randomized controlled trial (RCT) methodology, there are no RCTs on safety, particularly in relation to pregnancy, since it would be impossible to obtain ethics committee approval to conduct such a trial. The few papers available on aromatherapy in pregnancy and childbirth show wide variations in both research methodology and aromatherapy practice, and rely on an assumption that aromatherapy is "safe enough" for pregnant women, based largely on experiential reporting of benefits and lack of reporting of harm.

Homeopathy and energetic remedies

The German doctor, Samuel Hahnemann, developed homeopathy in the 18th century, and there are now several thousand homeopathic remedies in use around the world. Contemporary use of homeopathy is widespread; estimates suggest that up to 6 million US citizens self-administer the remedies on a regular basis (Clarke *et al.* 2015).

Hahnemann discovered that the principle of "treating like with like" was more effective and caused fewer side effects than many of the aggressive medical methods in use at the time, which often involved purging, bloodletting and other invasive techniques. Homeopathy is based on quantum physics and the concept of energy: remedies are produced by repeated dilution and succussion (vigorous shaking) of a substance, which, in its original form, may have been highly toxic. Remedies are derived from plants, animal substances (such as apis, from the honey bee), minerals (notably the tissue salts – see below) and occasionally from bacteria and viruses (known as nosodes and sometimes, although controversially, used as vaccination replacements). It has been shown that the action of succussion converts potential energy into kinetic energy, releasing the power of the substance into the water in which it is dissolved, and that the water has the ability to retain the memory of that substance (Ball 2004; Manzalini and Galeazzi 2019). When a person's individual symptom picture is matched to a specific homeopathically prepared medicine, the remedy is said to resonate with the body's innate energy, returning its own energetic vibration to the optimum 7.83 Hz level, thus facilitating a return to homeostatic balance. This can be understood by observing the side effects of substances in their original, undiluted form which, when used in homeopathic micro-doses, will treat the same symptoms. An example is coffee – excessive consumption of coffee may cause insomnia, agitation, headache and palpitations, but someone reporting the same symptoms could be treated homeopathically with a remedy called coffea, in which coffee has been highly diluted and succussed to release its therapeutic potential, that is, "treating like with like".

Homeopathy does not, therefore, work pharmacologically (chemically) and will not interact with conventional medicines or herbal remedies. However, since homeopathic remedies are highly diluted from the original substance, there is little, if anything, biologically active in the end product, which makes them chemically very fragile. This means that they can be inactivated by other stronger chemical, aromatic or energetic substances, including essential oils, coffee, peppermint, mint-flavoured toothpaste and chewing gum, X-rays, mobile telephones, microwave ovens and strong sunlight. Certain strong pharmaceutical drugs can also block the homeopathic action, including some analgesics, antacids, specific antibiotics, aspirin, steroids, laxatives, cough lozenges, decongestants and "deep heat" preparations for muscle pain.

Conversely, the argument amongst sceptics who do not understand the energetic mechanism of homeopathy is that the highly diluted nature of the remedies implies that they have "nothing in them" – and therefore they have no effect. This is not true, but unfortunately, despite its popularity, homeopathy is currently experiencing worldwide condemnation, primarily because it cannot be studied in the same way as herbal medicine or pharmaceutical research. There is minimal research using the "gold standard" RCT methodology because this does not fit the individualized precise prescribing required of homeopathy, a factor that contributes to its lack of acceptance by scientists (Mathie *et al.* 2017). When studies have been undertaken attempting to use randomized controlled, blinded methodology, results are either insignificant or inconclusive, leading scientists to reiterate their claim that homeopathy is ineffective. On the other hand, it must be acknowledged that either homeopathy does something and needs to be used judiciously, or it does nothing, in which case sceptics have nothing about which to be concerned.

The *WHO Traditional Medicine Strategy* (2013) reports that homeopathy is used in over 100 member states. Practitioner training varies from short six-month courses to two-year diploma programmes (UK), whilst in some countries homeopathy is integrated into four-year naturopathic degrees at both undergraduate and master's levels (USA and Germany). In South Africa, homeopaths have a similar status to medical practitioners following a five-year master's degree and a one-year internship.

Several countries are taking steps to regulate homeopathic practice more stringently and to restrict its use and the availability of remedies for self-administration to the public. The American FDA, which regulates medicines and herbal remedies, has required additional scrutiny of homeopathic remedies since 2017, and actively discourages the use of homeopathic preparations as a replacement for conventional vaccinations (FDA 2019). Canada took steps in 2015 to regulate homeopathic practice in ways similar to that of the conventional health professions (Ng 2020). In the UK, a campaign to discredit homeopathy has led to calls for a ban on its availability via the National Health Service (NHS), despite the fact that many medical doctors trained in homeopathy have previously provided thousands of homeopathic prescriptions for patients (Fernandez and Taylor 2019). Although homeopathy is one of the most popular complementary therapies in France, from 2021 the government will no longer reimburse the cost of homeopathic prescriptions via its health service, stating that there is no evidence of benefit (Scott 2019). Germany is the only EU country in which homeopathy is not restricted and continues to be used by many conventional healthcare professionals, including midwives. On the other hand, homeopathy is integrated into the conventional healthcare system in Mexico, while India has the largest proportion of homeopathic practitioners per head of population in the world (Abinavhavi 2014).

Tissue salts (sometimes called biochemical salts) are homeopathically prepared micro-doses of inorganic minerals found naturally in the human body. First formulated as medicinal products by Wilhelm Heinrich Schuessler in 1873, they are now incorporated as part of homeopathic practice. Schuessler (or Schußler) was a German medical doctor influenced by the teaching of Samuel Hahnemann and other homeopaths of the time. While mineral supplements replenish deficient mineral reserves in the body, tissue salts aim to support the body's healing processes by regulating electrolyte levels in the cells. Poor diet, stress, toxins and injury can block the homeostatic regulation of the cells, possibly leading to alterations in the sodium–potassium pump. It is theorized that tissue salts can boost the body's salt levels yet do not need to be broken down in the gastrointestinal tract before being assimilated, so that they facilitate the overall absorption of nutrients ingested in food. They are considered safe for pregnant women but should be taken selectively according to current symptoms. They are claimed to have no interactions with pharmacological medications, are non-addictive and, although most contain lactose, they are now also available without lactose for those with intolerances.

Flower essences, such as English Bach Flower Remedies, Australian Bush Flower Essences and the more obscure orchid essences and other traditional remedies using indigenous plants, are similarly energetic medicines although they are prepared differently from homeopathy and are used for different therapeutic purposes. Flower remedies are thought to tap into the energy of the sun, aiming to treat the emotional aspects of health and illness. It is claimed that they have no physical effects on the body, although the physiological impact of relieving emotional distress and trauma can be profound. The evidence base is almost nil, with just a few inconclusive studies investigating primarily Bach Rescue Remedy for stress (Muhlack *et al.* 2006; Resende *et al.* 2014; Rivas-Suárez *et al.* 2017; Wei Yang, Koo and Wang 2015). However, the remedies are available for public purchase and continue to have a following amongst homeopaths and consumers.

Traditional medicine systems

The WHO defines TM as "knowledge, skills and practices based on the theories, beliefs and experiences…indigenous to different cultures"

(WHO 2013). These include TCM and associated Eastern therapies, Indian Ayurveda and traditional African and Latin American medicine, although folk remedies are also used in parts of Europe and by aboriginal peoples in North and South America, Australasia and the Pacific region. All over the world TM focuses on a holistic body–mind–spirit approach, and incorporates the use of locally available plants, minerals and even animals. Treatment may also include massage and other manual techniques, dietary adaptations, exercises and meditation. Spiritual and religious rituals, chanting, prayers and music are also integrated in many TM systems; these are often shrouded in mystery and practised by shaman or witch doctors attempting to ward off the evil spirits believed to be responsible for ill health. Training varies, from observational work with experienced practitioners, as in African and many Latin American countries, to diploma and degree-level programmes for Chinese and Ayurvedic medicine, although there is also a worrying plethora of so-called "practitioner-level" courses that can be studied online at minimal expense. The WHO has accepted TCM and other traditional medical modalities into its global compendium, although this has not been universally welcomed (Hunt 2019).

TM is differentiated from CAM therapies and from folk medicine in that it is associated with discrete ethnic populations in defined geographical locations. TM usually involves a formal consultation with a local practitioner or healer, and is often integrated into a country's healthcare system, while folk remedies are passed on more informally by knowledgeable family members or friends, with little integration into local healthcare. For example, Asian systems of medicine have many ancient records with written philosophies and pharmacopoeia, and the Chinese government is committed to integrating TCM into conventional healthcare practice (Xinhua 2020). Conversely, African medicine is largely an oral tradition passed down from one generation to the next, although various governments across the continent acknowledge the significance of TM in their own regions.

The following are examples of TM:

- *Traditional Chinese medicine* (TCM) is based on the concept of meridians, energy lines that carry the body's life force (called Qi, pronounced "chee") and connect one part of the body to another. Excessive, deficient or stagnant flow of Qi causes disease to develop. Treatment incorporates acupuncture/acupressure, tuina massage, cupping, moxibustion, disciplined martial arts exercise such as Tai chi, diet and the use of indigenous herbs. Conventional medical education in China has, for some years, been required to include TCM in its undergraduate curricula (Hua *et al.* 2017).

- *Indian Ayurvedic medicine* uses the principles of the five universal elements of space, air, fire, water and earth; these combine to form three energetic life forces or doshas which dictate individual predisposition to disease. Treatment to restore dosha balance may involve blood purification, massage, enemas or laxatives, essential oils and local herbs. There has traditionally been cross-referral of patients between orthodox and complementary practitioners in India, and further legal changes to integrate the two systems more comprehensively have been made (Math *et al.* 2015).

- *Japanese kampo* is traditional herbal and mineral medicine based on that used in TCM and employing similar principles, whilst being largely plant-based medicines with fewer alternative techniques. Kampo medicines are classified by their pharmacological actions into tonic, purgative, heat clearing, expulsive, dispelling dampness and harmonization and regulation of Ki (the Japanese name for Qi). Kampo is widely used in the Japanese conventional medical system and is available as over-the-counter medication for self-administration; costs can be reimbursed by the government.

- *Traditional African medicine* incorporates indigenous herbalism and African spirituality. Herbal medications are prescribed not only for their pharmacological actions but also for their symbolic spiritual significance. Treatments may consist of fasting, dietary adaptations, massage, bathing and surgical procedures. More culturally significant methods may include bleed cupping, zootherapy (use of animals and animal products), magic and shamanism. Healers are seen not only as practitioners of medicine, but also as custodians of traditional practices, religious beliefs and customs, and as informal counsellors, social workers and psychologists (Mokgobi 2014). The WHO published guidelines for the registration of traditional African medicine some years ago, to facilitate greater integration into the healthcare provision across the continent, particularly in sub-Saharan Africa (WHO 2017).

- In *Latin America, shamans* are also an integral part of TM practice. They attempt to treat energetic and spiritual disharmony through astral or spiritual "journeys", tapping into human, animal and plant spirit energy and acting as a conduit to transfer this positive energy to the ill person. Indigenous plants are used for their spiritual and biological powers. Countries vary in respect of acceptance and regulation, but some, such as Brazil, have introduced legislation to ensure consistency of standards and to preserve local traditions (Carvalho *et al.* 2014).

Although there is emerging research on some elements of TM, notably on Chinese acupuncture and on many of the herbal remedies incorporated into the various systems around the world, the overall evidence base generally remains limited. There is considerable experience of using TM and empirical evidence of effectiveness abounds, but formal scientific research is more limited, particularly in respect of safety. In addition, where TM has been found to be unsuccessful, perhaps resulting in a person's death, this may in some cultures be attributed to spiritual aspects, such as offending the ancestors, or being in possession of evil spirits which prevent recovery from illness, rather than any acknowledgement of potential NR toxicity, mismanagement or delay in obtaining conventional medical treatment.

However, the globalization of TM raises implications for training and the competence of practitioners, as well as the regulation of the remedies used, to ensure safety. This is of particular concern when TMs are used in combination with conventional healthcare in developed countries, especially if taken surreptitiously without informing orthodox medical practition-ers. Many TM products are unregulated, even in their own countries of origin, and large amounts are now imported into developed countries, or are produced commercially and made available to purchase via the internet. Interestingly, in India, where Ayurvedic medicine is popular, the government took the unusual step in 2009 to proclaim almost 200,000 different traditional remedies and treatments as "public property" in a bid to prevent multinational companies from seeking commercial patents for them (Ramesh 2009).

TMs may occasionally be contaminated with toxic substances, either accidentally or sometimes intentionally – not with malicious intent but rather in the belief that certain additional substances enhance the therapeutic effect of the remedy. Specific remedies are banned in some countries due to irrefutable evidence of risk. An example of this is the herbal remedy, kava, which is banned in the UK, Germany, France, Switzerland, Australia and Canada due to concerns over its potential to cause liver toxicity (Pantano *et al.* 2016). It is still available in the USA although the issue remains contentious, and kava continues to be used in some cultures as a recreational herb (Kandola 2018; MHRA 2014).

TMs are sometimes made from animals and animal products, often involving endangered species. These include buffalo, leopard, reptiles, porcupine and pangolin in Africa, and clouded leopard, tiger, sea horse and bear amongst others in India, China and Mexico (Alonso-Castro 2014; Chakravorty, Meyer-Rochow and Ghosh 2011; Matthews-King 2019). Some products are imported from other countries, such as African rhinoceros horn used in China, Vietnam and other Far Eastern countries as an aphrodisiac and sexual stimulant (Hsu 2017).

The *WHO Traditional Medicine Strategy 2014–2023* (WHO 2013) aimed to "promote the safe and effective use of TM by regulating, researching and integrating TM products, practitioners and practice into health systems, where appropriate". By 2019, 170 countries (88 per cent of WHO member states) had formally developed policies, regulatory mechanisms and programmes to aid the integration of TM and CAM into national healthcare systems (WHO 2013).

Table 1 summarizes some of the features and the different mechanisms of action of the different types of NRs.

Table 1: Features of different NR modalities

	Derived from	Mechanism of action
Herbal remedies	Whole plants/parts of plants; includes oral, topical, inhalational, rectal, intravaginal, sometimes subcutaneous or intravenous use of essential oils	Pharmacological, i.e. chemical, mechanism of action – metabolized, utilized and excreted in the same way as drugs, irrespective of method of administration (although at different rates)
Aromatherapy	Essential oils extracted from different plants; administered by inhalation and topically via massage, creams, in water and as compresses	
Homeopathy	Plants, minerals, animal products, bacteria, viruses	Energetic remedies, mechanism of action not fully understood, based on quantum physics; not metabolized physically – NO pharmacological action
Tissue salts	Naturally occurring mineral salts used in homeopathic dilution, incorporated into homeopathic practice	
Flower remedies	Dilutions of plants, minerals, water prepared by exposure to sun or by boiling; aim to treat emotional aspects of health and illness	

	Derived from	**Mechanism of action**
Traditional medicines	Plants, minerals, animal products, bacteria; also manual therapies, nutritional and spiritual practices indigenous to different cultures around the world	Plant products act pharmacologically Other substances may work pharmacologically or energetically

2

The Use of Natural Remedies in Pregnancy and Childbirth

Surveys suggest that, in terms of herbal medicine, those most commonly used during pregnancy and birth, both in westernized and TM systems, appear to be aloe vera, chamomile, cranberry, echinacea, evening primrose, garlic, ginger, ginseng, peppermint, raspberry leaf and valerian (Cardoso and Amaral 2019; Kennedy *et al.* 2013). In addition, Bangladeshi women use lemon, prune, mustard oil and black seed (M. Ahmed *et al.* 2018), while Middle Eastern women favour thyme, sage, aniseed, cumin, fenugreek and olive oil (Al Essa *et al.* 2019; John and Shantakumari 2015). Aromatherapy is by far the most popular NR modality in developed countries, particularly by self-administration, but also professionally administered by independent practitioners and increasingly offered by midwives and doulas for labouring women.

Homeopathy and flower remedies tend to be less commonly used, or at least less commonly identified in research studies, surveys and authoritative publications. They are generally prescribed following professional consultation or self-administered by women already familiar with their therapeutic principles. The primary source of evidence for homeopathy in pregnancy appears to come from Germany where it is relatively well accepted alongside mainstream medical care (Münstedt *et al.* 2014), but no recent surveys identifying the incidence of use in pregnancy could be found. Homeopathic professional and regulatory organizations tend to expound the benefits of homeopathy in pregnancy, with advice to women on how to use the different remedies appropriately, rather than to pursue more academic research on the incidence of use or any potential adverse effects.

In a hierarchy of usage, popularity and safety, pregnant, labouring and postnatal women's access to NRs appears to be via various means, from self-administration to professional consultation, namely:

- Self-administration without consultation with a healthcare professional, either orthodox or complementary.

- Self-administration following advice from maternity care professionals who are not qualified in the relevant therapy.

- Administration by maternity care professionals who have some training but who are not fully qualified in the therapy.

- Administration by, or self-administration following consultation with, maternity care providers who are fully qualified in the NR modality.

- Consultation with a qualified complementary therapy practitioner with little or no post-registration education on application of the therapy to pregnancy, labour and the postnatal period.

- Consultation with an independent qualified medical herbalist or homeopath, or with a culturally approved traditional medicine practitioner, who prescribes appropriate remedies.

Self-administration of NRs

The self-administration of NRs is particularly prevalent amongst pregnant women in all cultures, with documented statistics coming from both developed and developing countries. Surveys in westernized countries in recent years have suggested that anything from 1 per cent to 87 per cent of expectant mothers may be self-administering NRs (Close *et al.* 2016; Hall, Griffiths and McKenna 2011; Sibbritt *et al.* 2014; Trabace *et al.* 2015). A large multinational study of almost 10,000 pregnant women from 23 countries investigated women's use specifically of herbal remedies (Kennedy *et al.* 2013). The study identified an average use of NRs of 29 per cent, the highest incidence being in Russia (69 per cent), Eastern Europe (51.8 per cent) and Australia (43.8 per cent). Another study found 23 per cent of Danish women self-administering herbal remedies, many on a daily basis (Volqvartz *et al.* 2019). In the USA, the number of pregnant women using CAM therapies in general appears to be around 67–68.5 per cent (Johnson *et al.* 2016; Strouss *et al.* 2014), although Kennedy *et al.* (2013) found only 26.6 per cent specifically using herbal or homeopathic remedies. Interestingly, an Australian study showed a relatively low use of herbal preparations, with the incidence of the most commonly used, raspberry leaf, evening primrose and spirulina, being under 5 per cent (Shand *et al*. 2016). This conflicts with earlier studies and is possibly not a true reflection of contemporary NR use by Australian women, especially given its popularity amongst midwives for use in labour (Frawley *et al*. 2015; Hall and Jolly 2014; Hall, McKenna and Griffiths 2012). In the Middle East, 72 per cent of pregnant women in Jordan use NRs, 56 per cent in Saudi Arabia, 49 per cent in Turkey and 22 per cent in Iran, while the increasing use of NRs for termination of pregnancy is causing concern (Al Essa *et al*. 2019; Ali-Shtayeh, Jamous and Jamous 2015; Kıssal, Çevik Güner and Batkın Ertürk 2017; Sabourian *et al*. 2016; Sattari *et al*. 2012). There appears to be less data on antenatal use of NRs in Latin America, although one Brazilian study indicated around 22 per cent of the general population using herbal medicines from garden plants, with women being the primary users (Zeni *et al*. 2017). Whilst NR use in pregnancy and labour is common across the world, it has, understandably, been shown to decrease during the postnatal period (Birdee *et al*. 2014).

However, as with studies of the non-pregnant population, the methodology used in many of these pregnancy-related surveys may not accurately reflect the real use of NRs. It is particularly difficult to elicit precise responses when women (and many health professionals) do not understand the differences between herbal, homeopathic and other types of natural remedies; often they do not recognize herbal teas as NRs, and nor do they appreciate the pharmacological nature of essential oils used in aromatherapy. Women may admit to self-administering a specific remedy yet do not take it correctly or in an appropriate therapeutic dose. They may seek aromatherapy treatment from a qualified practitioner but may identify more with the massage component (as a complementary therapy) than with the essential oils used (as NRs). Additionally, since many plants are used in both herbal medicine and homeopathy (same Latin names but prepared differently), surveys are dependent on women knowing the modality of the remedies they have used. This is because herbal remedies may be potentially toxic, yet the same plant prepared homeopathically and taken appropriately will potentially treat similar symptoms effectively without the pharmacological risk of toxicity. For example, blue cohosh (*Caulophyllum thalictroides*) is extremely toxic in its original herbal (pharmacological) form, whereas the highly diluted homeopathic (energetic) preparation, caulophyllum, from the same plant, can be a useful and safe remedy in labour.

Terminology and the way questions are asked of a study population may also elicit different responses. In a survey of 889 Scottish women, McLay *et al.* (2016) found that when a closed question was asked, such as "Have you used herbs/herbal medicines during pregnancy?", the positive response rate was just 4.3 per cent. When a checklist with named remedies was used, of those who originally answered "no", there were, in fact, as many as 39 per cent who had used one or more remedies. Allen *et al.* (2014) also raise this issue, in respect of both NRs and conventional drugs and other substances, such as alcohol. Similarly, asking women about their use of a specific NR for a specific condition, such as "ginger for sickness", may also be flawed: many women, especially in the UK, rely on commercially produced ginger biscuits, which contain very little ginger, rather than taking an appropriate therapeutic dose liable to be effective as an anti-emetic (see Tiran 2012).

In the developing world, traditional birth attendants (TBAs) embrace the use of indigenous plants to aid the birth process. Nalumansi, Kamatenesi-Mugisha and Anywar (2017) found that TBAs generally appear to have good knowledge on NRs, although Aziato and Omenyo (2018) disagree, suggesting that their lack of knowledge can threaten women's wellbeing. Recorded rates of NR use in Africa range from 20 per cent in Ghana to 62 per cent in Sierra Leone and up to 73 per cent in Ethiopia, but the actual percentage of women using NRs may be considerably higher (Jambo *et al.* 2018; James *et al.* 2018; Nyeko, Tumwesigye and Halage 2016; Laelago, Yohannes and Lemango 2016). On the Indian sub-continent, a systematic review of NR use in pregnancy across seven different Asian countries found an average use of 47 per cent (Ahmed *et al.* 2017), whereas in Bangladesh alone it was found to be up to 70 per cent (M. Ahmed *et al.* 2018). Hispanic communities in the Americas also have high antenatal herbal medicine use, with reportedly "good understanding" of their therapeutic purposes and the potential risks to their babies (Green *et al.* 2017).

Expectant mothers use NRs for many reasons, the most popular being to aid relaxation and ease antenatal discomforts, to prepare for the birth and to facilitate physiological progress in labour. Women's decisions to use NRs are possibly taken after analysing information from a variety of sources before drawing final conclusions (Barnes *et al.* 2018). Cultural norms and personal philosophies about health, as well as a desire to manage one's own health, are significant factors in women's choices in the western world (Peprah *et al.* 2019).

Many women self-administer NRs to resolve pregnancy symptoms, as well as incidental minor illnesses such as the common cold (M. Ahmed *et al.* 2018). Sometimes they resort to NRs for more specific medical or obstetric complications, such as urinary tract infections (Kennedy *et al.* 2013).

Yuvaci *et al.* (2019) revealed that almost 60 per cent of Turkish pregnant women with mental health issues were taking herbal teas, often concomitantly with prescribed antidepressants. This included some, such as St John's wort, which is contraindicated, both in pregnancy and in conjunction with antidepressant medication (Apaydin *et al.* 2016). There is a widespread misconception that NRs have fewer side effects and are more effective than medically prescribed drugs (James *et al.* 2018; Wolgast, Lindh-Åstrand and Lilliecreutz 2019). Arabiat *et al.* (2019), amongst other authorities, stress the need for more education of the public by health professionals on the dangers of NRs, although current lack of knowledge of midwives, doctors, doulas and other birth attendants first requires a concerted effort towards professional education (see below).

In developing countries, poverty is likely to be a motivator to self-administration of NRs for obstetric and gynaecological conditions, in preference to accessing costly medical advice, which may also involve long and arduous journeys (Jambo *et al.* 2018). In addition, societal and cultural reliance on local healers, especially in Africa, may exert an element of pressure on women to use TMs. Countries with male-dominated societies, coupled with paternalistic conventional health services, cause women to seek privacy, and the fear of possible mistreatment at the hands of male staff has also been suggested as a reason for self-administration, especially by women seeking termination of pregnancy (Gerdts *et al.* 2017). In many countries, cultural traditions require women to adopt a specific lifestyle during pregnancy, usually involving dietary and social restrictions and administration of herbal concoctions, with any obstetric complications being attributed to failure to comply with these customs; feelings of guilt lead to delay in seeking appropriate conventional treatment, possibly compounding the adverse effects of any continuing NR use (Riang'a, Nangulu and Broerse 2018).

The desire to expedite labour appears to be prevalent worldwide, with anything from raspberry leaf to elephant dung being used (Muñoz Balbontín *et al.* 2019; Panganai and Shumba 2016). Using herbs and homeopathy for the relief of pain and aiding progress in labour is also common, while breastfeeding women in many regions, particularly in developing countries, use herbs to stimulate lactation (James *et al.* 2019; Maonga *et al.* 2016) or to aid recovery from birth, as in China (Wang *et al.* 2018).

There is also a worrying use of NRs for neonates and infants. Women in many African countries, from Ethiopia to Nigeria to South Africa, use various local plants for infant colic and teething (Adane *et al.* 2020; Di Gaspero *et al.* 2019; Nwaiwu and Oyelade 2016). In the Middle East, 78 per cent of neonates with jaundice are given herbal remedies, despite the potential for many to be hepatotoxic, thus increasing the risk of kernicterus (Heydari *et al.* 2016). Even in the USA, 40 per cent of disadvantaged mothers in Houston, Texas, were found to be using honey pacifiers, despite honey being contraindicated in infants due to the risk of botulism from spores in the honey (Benjamins *et al.* 2013).

The use of natural remedies by maternity care professionals

Many midwives and birth workers advocate the use of NRs and other CAM therapies in their care of women during pregnancy and particularly in labour. In most cultures, the use of herbs and other NRs has been fundamental to childbirth for centuries, and many midwives and doulas want to return to the natural way of birthing that has been largely lost, especially in developed countries in which obstetrics presides over maternity care in a paternalistic, evidence-based, litigation-conscious manner.

There are, however, wide variations between countries in terms of education and training, practice, accountability lines and acceptance of NR use by midwives and other birth workers. Some maternity professionals are fully qualified in a therapy or have received maternity-specific training to enable them to use the therapy within strictly defined parameters to ensure safe practice. However, many more have little or no knowledge or understanding of NRs, particularly of the contraindications and precautions, correct doses, potential adverse effects and complications of inappropriate use, interactions with drugs or other orthodox treatments or their impact on maternal and fetal wellbeing and pregnancy and labour progress (Mollart, Stulz and Foureur 2019; Mollart *et al.* 2018). They are passionate about helping women to achieve physiological birth with as few interventions as possible but fail to acknowledge that any intervention, whether medical or "natural", is an interference in the intrinsic physiological process of pregnancy and childbirth.

Many midwives in Europe and Australia use essential oils combined with massage (Einion 2016; Hall, Griffiths and McKenna 2013), although most are not fully qualified in aromatherapy. Indeed, possession of a professional qualification in aromatherapy does not necessarily equip a midwife or doula to apply the principles of the therapy to its practice within maternity care. There is also an extremely worrying trend in some countries for midwives to undertake short maternity-specific courses in aromatherapy and then to attempt to train other colleagues, frequently without gaining practice to consolidate their own learning, and almost universally without adequate qualification or indemnity insurance to teach the subject (source: numerous communications with UK colleagues).

Whilst aromatherapy can offer a relaxing means of facilitating pregnancy and birth progress and is generally considered safe enough when used correctly, it could currently be deemed to be the most dangerous use of NRs in terms of inappropriate use, both by the women themselves but also when offered as an adjunct to midwifery or doula care. Women put their trust in maternity professionals to care for them safely, but this trust may be misplaced when midwives and doulas stretch their professional boundaries with the ill-informed use of aromatherapy. I have received numerous reports of pathological complications, sometimes attributable to the injudicious use of essential oils (source: communications with colleagues around the world).

In addition, the increasing number of aromatherapy studies undertaken by enthusiastic midwives with a poor understanding of essential oil safety is disturbing. A recent Iranian randomized, controlled, single-blinded study appeared to show the benefit of using lavender oil (type not specified) by inhalation for neonates undergoing painful investigative procedures such as venepuncture (Razaghi *et al.* 2020). However, essential oil use, especially by inhalation, is completely contraindicated in neonates due to rapid transfer across the blood–brain barrier and the need to metabolize the oils via an immature liver, risking serious toxicity (see Tiran 2016).

On the other hand, Italian midwives are proficient in the use of herbal remedies (Muñoz-Sellés, Vallès-Segalés and Goberna-Tricas 2013) and many obstetricians and midwives in Germany use homeopathy, although many feel the training is inadequate to ensure competence (Münstedt *et al.* 2014; Wiebelitz *et al.* 2013). Interestingly, since 2014, Belgian midwives have been permitted to use homeopathy after completion of a 50-hour course (Lombaerts and Vanthuyne 2018). Abedzadeh-Kalahroudi (2014) claimed that all midwives in the Middle East use NRs, although this statistic was not referenced, the type of NR was not specified and education of maternity providers on the safe use of NRs appears minimal and inconsistent. Many midwives and nurse-midwives in the USA use herbs in their practice, but most have less than five hours' training on the subject and many advise on, or administer, NRs without any specific training and often without medical knowledge or approval (Delmondao 2016; Dennehy *et al.* 2010).

In the developing world, where childbirth is often supported by unqualified TBAs, herbal medicines and other NRs are commonly incorporated into care, often with little, if any, formal training. Further, women's own use of NRs for general health, particularly to aid fertility, leads to continuing use during pregnancy, which appears to be condoned without question by TBAs (Kaadaaga *et al.* 2014). For most TBAs their experience and knowledge of NR use in pregnancy and birth is empirical, having been gained through apprenticeship with colleagues or as part of their own families' usage (Aziato and Omenyo 2018; Shewamene, Dune and Smith 2017). Some countries are beginning to formalize training programmes for TBAs to ensure greater safety for women (Hernandez, Oliveira and Sharazian 2017; Ohaja and Murphy-Lawless 2017), but the proportion of time, if any, spent on learning about the safety of NRs is not clear.

The interest and the desire to act as the mother's advocate amongst all maternity professionals is laudable but does pose some risks when maternity professionals are not fully qualified in the use of different NRs. As with the general public, many midwives, doulas and some obstetricians seem to believe that there is no risk from NRs, usually because they do not appreciate the mechanism of action, notably of pharmacological herbal remedies, including essential oils used in aromatherapy.

3

Risks of Natural Remedies in Pregnancy and Birth

Whilst there are undoubtedly many benefits from using NRs in day-to-day life, especially for reproductive health and wellbeing, many consumers and health professionals fail to understand that "natural" does not mean these remedies are automatically safe; conversely, it does not mean that they are inactive. The greatest concern relates to herbal medicines, from both indigenous plants and TMs, mainly because these have pharmacological effects, are generally unlicensed and are easily accessible by the public. There are significant risks to women using NRs and TMs, especially during labour and when used in combination with conventional drugs.

Nothing is without risk. All NRs have physiological effects that may be either positive or negative depending on how they are used. However, it is important not to leap to conclusions about the potential adverse effects of NRs through lack of understanding of phytochemistry and energetic principles and the factors that may affect them. Risk needs to be put in context rather than being seen as absolute. NRs may indeed be safe enough, when prescribed by appropriately trained professionals with dual knowledge of both the specific modality and its application to pregnancy and birth. No single pharmaceutical drug is appropriate or safe for every individual with the same symptoms, and this principle also applies to the use of NRs. Drugs are prescribed following an assessment and careful decision-making about the most effective and safest treatment, with close supervision and evaluation of its effects. Professional practitioners of the various NRs also follow this process, but this is not the case when women decide to self-prescribe NRs; indeed, what is appropriate for one woman is not necessarily safe for another.

Sceptics claim that any benefits of NRs are due to the placebo effect, particularly in relation to the poorly understood energetic medicines, but it must be acknowledged that a placebo can be a powerful entity in its own right. On the other hand, doctors are quick to blame "quack medicine" when an individual taking NRs develops untoward reactions, even though the symptoms may be unrelated to the remedies. Others criticize the apparent lack of evidence for both effectiveness and safety, although this is not a reason to reject consideration of risk: in some respects lack of evidence can pose more risk in human terms because healthcare professionals may choose to ignore these "alternative" remedies and may not be alert to the possibility of detrimental effects. Indeed, lack of evidence of the potential for harm is not the same as proof of safety.

There are several types of risk from NRs that may impact on maternal or fetal health and the progress of pregnancy and labour, including:

- Direct and indirect adverse effects of NRs.

- Potentially toxic effects of NRs.

- Interactions between NRs and drugs or other NRs.

- Specific adverse effects of NRs on pregnancy and labour.

- Contraindications and precautions to use of NRs in pregnancy and childbirth.

Direct and indirect adverse effects of NRs

Stub *et al.* (2016) consider direct risk in which NRs cause physiological complications through toxicity (see below), and indirect risk as a result of poor communication between patients and healthcare providers (human factors).

Indirect risk may arise from:

- Women's non-disclosure of self-administration of NRs without professional consultation.

- Women's non-disclosure of NR use prescribed by an independent qualified practitioner.

- Professional prescription of NRs by a qualified practitioner without communication with maternity care providers.

- Informal non-documented advice on NRs by well-meaning but ill-informed maternity professionals.

- Use of NRs integrated into conventional maternity care by maternity professionals without adequate knowledge.

Maternity professionals may be unaware of women's use or may fail to recognize the impact of NRs on a mother's or baby's condition or the progress of pregnancy or birth. Numerous surveys reveal that patients almost universally fail to offer information voluntarily to their healthcare providers about their use of NRs or other CAM therapies (Allen *et al.* 2014; Davis *et al.* 2012; James *et al.* 2018; Johny, Cheah and Razitasham 2017; Kelak, Cheah and Safii 2018). This non-disclosure occurs both in developed and developing countries, even when patients are being treated for serious medical conditions (Adane *et al.* 2020; Bahall 2017; Henson *et al.* 2017; Peprah *et al.* 2019). Non-disclosure applies both to the use of NRs that have been prescribed by an independent practitioner and to women's self-administration without appropriate professional advice.

Despite the incidence of NR use being higher amongst the pregnant population than most others, expectant mothers may think that it is not necessary for maternity carers to know about their use of NRs, or that they are not interested. They may fear having their views disparaged and their preferences disregarded. They may perceive conventional healthcare professionals as not knowing enough about NRs, or may not feel comfortable sharing information about their intended or actual use (Johny *et al.* 2017; Johny, Whye and Safii 2018). In developed countries, some women may be comfortable using NRs such as homeopathy, perhaps having used them for many years, and do not consider it important to inform their maternity care providers. Others commence self-administration of NRs in pregnancy as a replacement for medical drugs that they know are discouraged. This is commonly without any consultation with health professionals: women appear to gain most of their initial information on NRs from friends and family, with the obvious risk that it is not always accurate or comprehensive enough to ensure safe use (Kissal *et al.* 2017; Pallivalapila *et al.* 2015).

The huge rise in the self-administration of NRs by the public, particularly when accessing potentially incorrect, incomplete or contradictory online information, frequently leads people to use NRs inappropriately, risking potentially harmful effects. Surveys suggest that women are largely unaware of the possible harmful effects of NRs (Barišić *et al.* 2017; Barnes *et al.* 2018; Bettiol *et al.* 2018). There is widespread acknowledgement amongst both conventional and CAM authorities that more research is needed on the safety of NRs and that women must be encouraged to disclose their use, whether through professional consultation with the relevant practitioners or from self-administration (Boltman-Binkowski 2016; Bruno *et al.* 2018). Failure to do so may, at the very least, confuse the presenting symptom picture or complicate the woman's medical or obstetric condition or, in extreme cases, lead to serious toxicity and even fetal or maternal death.

Conversely, whilst most maternity professionals do not consciously enquire about women's use of CAM therapies and NRs, many expectant mothers are given superficial advice about the use of NRs by well-meaning midwives, doctors or doulas, often incorrectly (Al Essa *et al.* 2019; Barnes *et al.* 2018; Kennedy *et al.* 2013; Koc, Topatan and Saglam 2012; personal communications with colleagues). Indeed, recommendations to take herbal remedies that are contraindicated in pregnancy are three times more likely to come from a maternity professional than from an informal source (Kennedy *et al.* 2016). Maternity professionals generally know very little about NRs, but there is an increasingly urgent need for greater awareness as the incidence of use amongst pregnant women escalates exponentially.

Contemporary medical and midwifery education in most countries does not include the subject of "complementary therapies" or "natural remedies" as part of the pre-registration curriculum. In midwifery, those universities and other training establishments that do include the subject usually focus on the enjoyable relaxation effects of therapies such as massage or aromatherapy. Little coverage is given to the significant use of NRs by women in the preconception, antenatal, intrapartum or postpartum periods. In both midwifery and medical education, if an introduction to CAM is included, either at undergraduate or postgraduate level, this mostly explores the benefits as a means of increasing advocacy for women, and frequently fails to balance the subject with in-depth exploration of potential hazards and interactions with conventional care, based on contemporary evidence.

Some midwives and doctors seem either to disparage or reject NRs, effectively abdicating any responsibility to provide women with information through their own lack of knowledge. Conversely, others allow their enthusiastic advocacy for natural methods, and a desire to help women, to influence the advice they give. This can be evidenced amongst midwives in many parts of the world (Adib-Hajbaghery and Hoseinian 2014; Koc *et al.* 2012; Stewart *et al.* 2014). Occasionally, too, some doulas may use NRs clandestinely, especially in labour, perhaps in an attempt to maintain the balance of power between themselves and midwives or doctors (Stevens *et al.* 2011). Virtually all authors conclude that midwives, maternity nurses, doulas, medical staff and pharmacists need more education on the safe use of

NRs in pregnancy and childbirth, but despite the valiant efforts of specialist authorities on the subject, this is still very far from being made universally available.

Conversely, women may consult a qualified practitioner of herbal medicine, homeopathy, aromatherapy or TM during their pregnancies. Whilst western medical herbalists and homeopaths cover reproductive health as part of their pre-registration training, the subject of pregnancy – and particularly labour – is a post-registration aspect of aromatherapy and other complementary modalities. For many therapies, it is not mandatory to undertake specialist training on reproductive health in order to work with pregnant and newly birthed mothers. Further, post-registration maternity training is often superficial and poorly applied to pregnancy, birth and postnatal anatomy and physiology. Training is often provided by a therapy tutor with an interest in working with pregnant clients, or by a therapy tutor accompanied by a midwife, both of whom may be experts in their own field but who have limited understanding of how the two elements marry together.

There is little, if any, communication between complementary practitioners and conventional maternity professionals, protagonists on both sides of the health divide possibly believing that their particular expertise is sufficient to ensure safety for their clients. Poor interprofessional communication may also be due to medical dominance and a lack of appreciation of the roles of complementary practitioners (Nguyen *et al.* 2019). McIntyre *et al.* (2020) suggest that the use of a designated tool to ensure sharing of information between conventional and complementary practitioners could reduce the risks associated with non-disclosure by individuals. Further, this would ensure discussion on the impact of one modality with the other and enable better understanding of the impact of and interaction between orthodox and complementary care.

Disclosure of NR use requires two-way communication in order to avoid indirect adverse effects. This may be interaction between pregnant women and midwives and doctors, or between doulas and midwives, or between complementary practitioners and maternity professionals. At the very least, medical and midwifery staff should routinely ask expectant mothers about their use of NRs and document their answers in the women's maternity records. The question may need to be asked at the first antenatal appointment, in the third trimester when birth preparation is discussed and again in early labour to elicit what the mother may have taken already to aid progress and ease pain. Whilst the use of NRs tends to be less in the postnatal period, healthcare providers working with breastfeeding women should also be alert to their possible use of NRs. Conventional maternity staff may not know all the answers to the women's questions, but taking note of their self-administration or prescriptions from independent practitioners at least highlights the possibility of interactions and adverse effects if a woman's condition deteriorates, particularly if no other reason can be found. An example of this would be the admission of a woman in apparently idiopathic preterm labour, who may have injudiciously been using NRs such as raspberry leaf, evening primrose or clary sage oil to prepare for birth but which prematurely stimulate contractions.

Zheng *et al.* (2019) go so far as to suggest the need for communication between governmental and professional bodies, and clinical, educational and research organizations, to enable maternity providers to inform women about the currently available evidence of efficacy and safety of NRs and to direct them to reliable sources of information. They also advocate the need for collaboration with patient support groups to educate those working with pregnant, labouring and breastfeeding women.

Many NRs cause unpleasant responses. These reactions may be anticipated or unanticipated and are related to both correct and incorrect administration (doses, mode, duration, etc.). Adverse reactions to NRs may exacerbate the presenting symptoms and tend to persist until treatment is discontinued or modified. Alternatively, a remedy may have no beneficial effect and the presenting symptoms may worsen; this is not technically an adverse reaction to the remedy but rather a consequence of the delay in obtaining appropriate medical treatment due to a misplaced reliance on the NR.

Appropriate prescription of NRs following an in-depth consultation with a knowledgeable, experienced medical herbalist, homeopath, aromatherapist or qualified TM practitioner is far less likely to result in adverse effects due to erroneous use. However, given that the majority of pregnant and childbearing women will be cared for by doctors, midwives, doulas and other birth workers, and the fact that huge numbers of expectant mothers are self-administering NRs, the potential for harmful effects is much greater.

There are several types of physiological reactions that may occur with NRs:

- Normal healing reactions to correctly administered homeopathic/energetic remedies.

- Abnormal reverse provings to incorrectly administered homeopathic/energetic remedies.

- Adverse reactions caused by direct side effects to pharmacological herbs and drugs.

- Indirect adverse reactions to pharmacological herbs and drugs.

A *healing reaction*, sometimes called an aggravation or Jarisch-Herxheimer reaction, is a normal, anticipated reaction to homeopathy or other energy-based medicines such as flower remedies (and also occurs with other CAM modalities such as reflexology or acupuncture). The effects usually occur at the start of a correctly prescribed course of homeopathic treatment; inappropriate prescribing either produces no reaction or a reverse proving (see below). The individual may experience a temporary, relatively mild aggravation of the presenting symptoms, new symptoms may develop, such as skin irritation, or old symptoms may re-emerge, for example discomfort at a healed fracture site. This is seen as the body attempting to expel toxic or antagonistic metabolites in response to appropriate treatment that aims to facilitate regeneration. Symptoms occur during this process because the body is attempting to cleanse itself of existing toxins faster than they can be eliminated: the higher the toxin levels, the slower the regeneration, and the healing reaction will therefore be more exacting. Indeed, lack of a healing reaction to a correctly prescribed remedy may infer that the remedy has not yet been effective in treating the person's condition. Previously, some CAM practitioners termed this effect a "healing crisis", but this implies a problematic response, whereas a significant healing reaction is welcomed as a mark that the correct treatment has been given and the body is reacting well to it. Unfortunately, the uninitiated may erroneously believe these anticipated healing reactions are "side effects" caused by the NRs.

Negative responses to homeopathic and energy-based remedies occur through incorrect use or overdose. If a homeopathic remedy is administered inappropriately, either the right remedy taken for too long, in too high a dose or too frequently, or the wrong remedy is used, a *reverse proving* occurs in which the person develops the symptoms that the incorrectly administered remedy is intended to treat. This means that, not only are the presenting symptoms and their cause not treated, but also new symptoms are superimposed on the original ones. An example sometimes seen in newly birthed mothers incorrectly taking homeopathic arnica to reduce perineal bruising is a reverse proving in which systemic bruising develops (usually due to taking tablets too frequently). It should be noted here that, since homeopathic remedies do not act chemically, increased doses are generally achieved by increasing the frequency of administration, not by increasing the number of tablets at each administration. Further, extremely frequent administration of remedies is usually applied only to very acute situations – for example, a primary postpartum haemorrhage may require a remedy to be administered every 30 seconds. Correct administration of homeopathic arnica after a normal delivery would involve taking one tablet of an appropriate potency (commonly 30c) no more than four times daily for a maximum period of four days.

A reverse proving is an adverse reaction to a homeopathic remedy, not a side effect, since homeopathy does not act pharmacologically. There is no interaction of homeopathic remedies with other substances such as drugs or herbal medicines, although some prescribed medication can antidote (that is, inactivate) the remedies because they are chemically stronger. The easiest way to reduce the effects of inappropriate administration is simply to stop taking the remedy; unlike the metabolism of herbal remedies and drugs, there is no risk of negative reactions from sudden withdrawal, nor is there a continuation of pharmacological action until complete excretion of waste products.

It is, however, necessary to identify the precise nature of any untoward effects occurring during treatment with homeopathy. In Posadzki et al.'s systematic review of homeopathy (2013), 30 patients were reported as experiencing adverse reactions which were deemed to be "directly attributable" to the homeopathic prescription, while a further 8 suffered negative effects as a result of substitution of conventional medical care with homeopathy. However, their assertion that "homeopathy has the potential to harm patients…in both direct and indirect ways" fails to take account of those relatively minor reactions occurring in response to an appropriately prescribed dose of a remedy, that is, a normal healing response. Further, the authors provide an astonishingly comprehensive list of life-threatening conditions apparently "caused" by taking homeopathic medicines, including acute pancreatitis, bladder cancer, cardiac arrest and the need for renal dialysis. There seems to be little acknowledgement of the non-pharmacological nature of homeopathy and a reliance on the authors of the reviewed papers correctly identifying the adverse events as being related solely to homeopathy. Furthermore, failure to seek medical advice in favour of homeopathy cannot be viewed as an adverse effect of the homeopathy in particular: patients could self-administer any other substance instead of seeking medical advice, including over-the-counter drugs, yet this course of action would not be classified as an "adverse effect" of the drugs. In addition, some sweeping conclusions were drawn about the dangers of homeopathy, a fact that was challenged by several medical homeopaths in subsequent papers (Johnson 2014; Tournier, Roberts and Viksveen 2013; Walach, Lewith and Jonas 2013).

However, since 2011 the US FDA has received over 400 reports of adverse reactions in infants given homeopathic teething granules or gels (Abbassi 2017). These included infants suffering convulsions, dyspnoea, drowsiness, coma and gastrointestinal complaints, as well as 10 deaths thought to be directly attributable to the remedies. The FDA advised parents not to use the products, and several companies have voluntarily withdrawn stock from sale; one company issued a recall on a homeopathic teething product found to contain inconsistent amounts of belladonna. This is therefore not an error in clinical prescribing but an error in commercial preparation of the remedy, but this issue is likely to be another setback for the acceptance of homeopathy. It is also possible that some parents used the remedies inappropriately, triggering reverse provings. Unfortunately, as with the adverse effects of herbal medicines, problems with homeopathy most likely occur with incorrect use due to poor knowledge and lack of understanding of the mechanism of action.

Herbal medicines, aromatherapy essential oils and many traditional remedies contain significant amounts of pharmacologically active ingredients, some of which are potentially toxic and liable to cause negative, sometimes serious, reactions. The term "adverse reactions" is often used to describe all negative responses to pharmacological substances, but technically, there is a difference between side effects and adverse effects.

Side effects are defined as undesirable, but sometimes anticipated, reactions that can be directly related to the chemical action of the remedy, usually from administration of a normal dose, perhaps over a prolonged period of time. Side effects are generally new symptoms arising shortly after commencing treatment, but they tend to resolve with time as the individual becomes accustomed to the causative agent. Side effects are generally less likely to occur with appropriately prescribed herbal remedies than with pharmaceutical drugs, in which a single active ingredient has been isolated from the plant and synthesized in order that a commercial patent can be obtained. An example would be aspirin, a side effect of which is gastritis. Its active component, salicylate, is derived from salicin in the bark of the willow tree. When taken correctly as a herbal remedy, other constituents in the willow bark act synergistically to suppress the gastric irritant effects that occur with salicylate in isolation.

Strictly, *adverse effects* are unexpected, detrimental indirect interactions with other chemicals, whether naturally occurring in the body, as with hormones and enzymes, or from chemicals entering the body, such as drugs, foods, recreational substances and environmental toxins. Additional factors impacting on the tendency to develop adverse reactions to drugs and NRs include gender, age, genetic predisposition, current state of health, tendency to allergies and concomitant administration of multiple pharmacological agents.

Since 2012, the EU definition of "adverse reactions" has included negative effects due to error (inclusion or omission), misuse or abuse, as well as reactions to unlicensed medicines. For the purposes of this book, the term "adverse effects" is used throughout the alphabetical listing that follows to denote any negative responses, whether they are direct side effects or indirect adverse reactions.

Izzo *et al.* (2016) acknowledge the potential for adverse effects from NRs, identifying pregnancy, birth and childhood as particular risk periods. Individuals may experience adverse reactions or side effects to a named remedy, or to specific constituents within it. Ingestion, and dermal, respiratory, rectal, intravaginal or intravenous exposure, can contribute to adverse effects, primarily but not solely when administered in therapeutic doses. Effects may be acute or chronic; some effects may be immediate, or they emerge after prolonged use, for example carcinogenesis. Overdose or sudden withdrawal can cause deleterious reactions. Toxic compounds, either naturally occurring or from additives, such as mercury, lead or arsenic sometimes found in imported TMs, may also cause potentially lethal effects (Angelon-Gaetz *et al.* 2018; Sensi *et al.* 2019).

Adverse effects of all types are more likely to occur when women self-administer NRs without appropriate consultation with a qualified practitioner. Lack of knowledge poses a significantly increased risk of adverse reactions from NRs that are known to be contraindicated in pregnancy or birth, or that should not be used with certain medical conditions or treatments. Volqvartz *et al.* (2019) found that almost a quarter of pregnant women in Denmark were regularly administering herbal remedies, particularly ginger and liquorice. This is despite ginger having proven anticoagulant effects and the high salt content of liquorice being associated with hypertension, therefore requiring avoidance or caution in pregnancy. A review of Jordanian women's use of medicinal plants to aid conception found that many of the herbal remedies had antifertility actions (non-implantation, early miscarriage) rather than the presumed fertility-enhancing effects (Akour *et al.* 2016). In both developed and developing countries there is a concerning lack of knowledge amongst women about the correct doses, contraindications and precautions related to NRs and the need to avoid them altogether when taking prescribed drugs (Ghazali, Bello and Kola-Mustapha 2019; Smeriglio, Tomaino and Trombetta 2014).

Some authorities go so far as to suggest that health professionals should actively discourage women from using NRs during pregnancy and birth because the possibility of adverse effects is greater than any benefit that may be derived from the remedies (Muñoz Balbontín *et al.* 2019), although this may exacerbate the indirect risk of non-disclosure. Whilst there is little formal research of specific obstetric risks from the injudicious use of NRs, there is growing empirical evidence of adverse reactions. Indeed, the self-use of contraction-promoting NRs, such as raspberry leaf, blue cohosh, castor oil, evening primrose and clary sage, before or during medical induction of labour, has been shown to increase the incidence of obstetric complications and fetal distress, in some cases by as much as 55 per cent (Dante *et al.* 2014; Panganai and Shumba 2016; Zamawe *et al.* 2018; personal communications with colleagues).

Table 2 summarizes the different reactions to NRs.

Table 2: Types of reactions to natural remedies

Healing reaction	Normal, anticipated, desirable elimination of toxic metabolites from administration of energy-based remedies such as homeopathy; seen as a requisite precursor to self-healing and resolution of presenting problem. Temporary, usually occurring at start of treatment; treatment should be continued
Reverse proving	Adverse, undesirable reaction to inappropriate or incorrect administration of a homeopathic remedy, triggering symptoms that the incorrectly administered remedy is intended to treat. Symptom picture is compounded by failure to treat with the correct remedy, with superimposed symptoms caused by the incorrect remedy. Treatment with the offending remedy should be discontinued
Side effect	Undesirable, possibly predictable, direct reactions to the specific remedy or to specific chemical components, often with administration of normal therapeutic doses; effects usually reduce as body becomes accustomed to remedy. Treatment may be continued but should be reviewed and discontinued if side effects outweigh the benefit of the remedy
Adverse reaction	Unintended, often unexpected indirect effects of pharmacological agents in combination with intrinsic or extrinsic chemicals entering the body; often dependent on individual susceptibility
	OR Negative unexpected reactions to incorrect administration, often due to lack of knowledge; may be unrecognized through women's non-disclosure; may cause life-threatening toxicity of major organs or body systems. Treatment should be discontinued, gradually or immediately (depends on precise remedy)
No effect	Pharmacological agents – may be due to non-therapeutic dose or placebo effect
	Energy-based remedies – may be due to administration of incorrect remedy or may be significant in terms of the healing process – further/different treatment is needed to trigger an appropriate healing reaction

Potentially toxic effects of NRs

Adverse effects of NRs, as with drugs, are usually mild to moderate, such as allergic reactions or gastrointestinal effects. Prompt recognition of anticipated symptoms and discontinuation of the remedy can minimize any exacerbation of direct side effects that may occur. True unexpected adverse reactions can, however, occasionally cause life-threatening toxicity, especially if there is a delay in the recognition of symptoms and continued use of the NRs. Acute toxicity is defined as the toxic effects of exposure, usually to a single or large dose, whereas chronic toxicity occurs with prolonged exposure, sometimes over months or years. In some cases, the toxicity potential of some chemical agents declines with time as the substances degrade, but with others, such as essential oils, degradation in the form of oxidation may increase the risk of adverse effects. Systems particularly affected include the hepatic, renal, cardiac, haematological or neurological systems. For clarification, it should be noted in the discussion that follows that the issue of toxicity applies primarily to pharmacologically active NRs rather than to homeopathic or other energetic medicine modalities.

Gastrointestinal effects such as transient diarrhoea may result from taking any herbal remedy, not simply laxative herbs. Nausea and vomiting, heartburn, indigestion and oesophageal reflux, abdominal pain and bloating may also develop. More prolonged effects can lead to dehydration, electrolyte disturbance, oesophageal varices and other serious systemic conditions. Common herbs that may cause gastrointestinal effects include aloe vera, cascara, senna and St John's wort, but many others will initiate symptoms in susceptible people. Upper gastrointestinal tract allergic reactions from the oral administration of some NRs include mouth irritation and ulceration, with swelling of the lips and tongue. Causative examples include celery, aniseed, pineapple, coriander, cumin, fennel, parsley, dandelion and hibiscus, ingested either as foods or herbal remedies. Direct lower gastrointestinal effects are, however, less common than the indirect stomach and intestinal symptoms resulting from toxicity to other systems.

Integumentary adverse reactions include skin or mucous membrane irritation, erythema, blistering, heat and inflammation. With prolonged use, eczema and psoriasis can develop. Some NRs may affect the skin irrespective of the method of administration. Skin sensitivity is the easiest adverse reaction to detect as it usually occurs during or shortly after topical administration (contact dermatitis or primary sensitivity) (Pokladnikova et al. 2016); dermal reactions to ingested NRs may take longer to develop (secondary sensitivity). Topical use of essential oils, such as tea tree and eucalyptus, can trigger primary sensitivity, notably but not exclusively when the oil has oxidized.

Other essential oils may be rich in phenols, including clove, cinnamon, basil, thyme and aniseed. NRs that may trigger secondary skin reactions include poison ivy, cannabis oil, castor bean, celery, chrysanthemum, echinacea, garlic, ginkgo biloba and Panax ginseng, as well as combination products (Palanisamy, Haller and Olson 2003). Phototoxicity, in which direct exposure of the skin to strong sunlight causes burning, blistering and pain, may result from the use of NRs such as St John's wort or furocoumarin-rich essential oils including bergamot, bitter orange, carrot seed, lemon and lime.

Vaginal steaming with herbs, popularly used after childbirth by indigenous peoples in southern Africa, Thailand, Indonesia and parts of Latin America, may impact on the mucus membranes and vaginal flora, predisposing the woman to vaginal irritation and infections (Hull *et al.* 2011; van der Helm *et al.* 2019). Similarly, injudicious long-term use of herbal and coffee enemas may damage the rectal mucosa (Lee *et al.* 2020; Prasad *et al.* 2012).

Respiratory reactions, including dyspnoea, rhinitis, asthma, hay fever, cough and respiratory arrest, can occur with both inhalational use – as with essential oil vapours – or with oral use. Some individuals are sensitive to specific plant groups and may experience a variety of allergic respiratory reactions from oral, dermal or inhalational exposure. Those who are allergic to the Asteraceae/Compositae family, which includes daisies, chrysanthemums, marigolds, ragwort and others, are particularly vulnerable to dyspnoea, hay fever, asthma and anaphylaxis. Occupational exposure to the dust from herbal preparations can also impair respiratory function (Golec *et al.* 2005).

Renal toxicity – the negative impact of NRs on the renal system – may only become apparent when there is severe kidney impairment. In pregnancy, variations in renal function may be deemed to be obstetric-related before any association with NR use is made. For example, the salt content of liquorice root consumption may cause fluid retention, hypertension and altered serum electrolytes (Asif 2012), possibly masquerading as severe pre-eclampsia. Cranberry and other herbs raise oxalate levels, increasing the risk of renal calculi, even though cranberry is often used to treat urinary tract infections and cystitis. Examples of common herbs that may adversely impact on the renal system include blue cohosh, cat's claw, ginkgo biloba, horsetail, juniper berry, ma huang, pennyroyal, stinging nettle, St John's wort and yohimbe. Concern has also been expressed about the potential renal toxicity resulting from the use of Chinese medicinal herbs (Yang *et al.* 2018).

Liver toxicity is a very real risk of many herbal remedies administered orally, or even via the skin, respiratory tract or other routes, since the liver is the primary organ of metabolism and detoxification. Some herbs, such as agrimony, are significantly hepatotoxic (Cho *et al.* 2018), whereas others, for example echinacea, may only cause problems in susceptible individuals following prolonged use. An online Editorial from *The Lancet* (2018) suggested that the incidence of liver toxicity from herbal supplements has risen steadily in the last decade and now accounts for 20 per cent of all drug-induced cases in the USA, and an unbelievable 70 per cent in Singapore and South Korea. Andrade *et al.* (2018) suggest that, as women are more likely than men to resort to herbal medicines, they are statistically more prone to hepatotoxicity and therefore at greater risk of needing liver transplants or of dying from liver disease.

Early signs of developing hepatic pathology may be non-specific, possibly delaying recognition of NRs as the causative factor. Symptoms include tiredness and lethargy, nausea, vomiting, abdominal cramps and diarrhoea, as well as dermal hypersensitivity and rashes. Some of these may be misinterpreted as an exacerbation of physiological antenatal disorders until other signs such as fever and jaundice follow. However, the symptom picture can be similar to that of general hepatic disease, and it is essential that midwives and obstetricians are alert to the possibility of women ingesting NRs that may precipitate adverse hepatic reactions. This is especially significant in the event of suspected obstetric cholestasis. Many herbal remedies used in Chinese, Ayurvedic and Japanese kampo medicine are reported to cause hepatotoxicity, notably in those containing multiple ingredients, although this may sometimes be due to contaminants rather than the specific remedies (Iwata *et al.* 2016; Liu *et al.* 2018). Indeed, Teschke and Eickhoff (2015) call for herbal remedies to be reclassified globally as drugs since the risks of hepatotoxicity are significant. Examples of herbs that are potentially hepatoxic include: black cohosh, borage, echinacea, fennel, greater celandine, green tea, juniper berry, kava, marjoram, nutmeg, pennyroyal, skullcap and valerian.

Although less common than hepatic or renal adverse effects, *cardiovascular toxicity* can be serious, and mostly involves changes in cardiac electrical conduction or damage to cardiac muscle function, leading to inefficient circulation of the blood. Symptoms of developing cardiotoxicity include oedema, tachycardia, a dry non-productive cough, weakness and vertigo. Some plant medicines have a direct effect on the heart and cardiovascular system, such as deadly nightshade, liquorice and mandrake. A systematic review by Jalili *et al.* (2013) found hypertensive effects of herbs such as bitter orange, blue cohosh, dong quai, ginkgo, ginseng, liquorice, ma huang, pennyroyal, senna, St John's wort and yohimbe, whilst others may reduce blood pressure, including cat's claw, garlic and kudzu (Tabassum and Ahmad 2011). This means that these herbs would be contraindicated in women with hypertension, particularly those taking medication, and caution should be employed by women with low blood pressure who take hypotensive herbs. Cardiovascular symptoms may also arise from the adverse effects on other systems, usually with excessive or prolonged use of specific remedies.

Neurotoxicity – toxins in some NRs can affect the peripheral and/or central nervous systems, causing damage to the neurons and impacting on neurological activity. Symptoms include anxiety, depression, confusion and behavioural changes, weakness and numbness of the limbs, loss of bodily functions with altered reflexes, impaired vision, headaches and sexual dysfunction. Toxic effects on the autonomic nervous system are significant and can affect the cardiovascular, respiratory, gastrointestinal and endocrine systems. Potentially neurotoxic herbs include opium, cannabis, deadly nightshade, henbane, hemlock, yellow vine and angel's trumpet. Even popular essential oils such as peppermint and tea tree can, when taken orally, cause unconsciousness, convulsions and other near-fatal effects (Hammer *et al.* 2006; Nath, Pandey and Roy 2012).

Anticoagulant and antiplatelet effects of herbal remedies and TMs can also be significant. Many herbs are known to have substantial amounts of chemical constituents such as salicylates that affect clotting factors or platelet aggregation. Early effects may include widespread bruising of the skin, increased clotting time for minor injuries or, in pregnancy, excessive bleeding of the gums and apparently idiopathic vaginal bleeding. Medical herbalists have long been cautious when prescribing remedies for patients on anticoagulant therapy such as heparin or warfarin, or taking other medicines or therapeutic doses of herbs with a similar action, such as aspirin or ginger (Abebe 2019; Choi, Oh and Jerng 2017; Stoddard *et al.* 2015). Indeed, the evidence for the anticoagulant effect of numerous herbal remedies, coupled with the potential central nervous system depressant effects of some, has led anaesthetists to advise patients due for elective surgery to discontinue all herbal remedies for at least two weeks prior to surgery (Kam, Barnett and Douglas 2019). This would be good advice for women booked for elective Caesarean section or other planned surgery during pregnancy. Similarly, women requiring dental surgery or extractions during pregnancy should be advised to inform their dentists prior to the procedures. Some examples of herbs known to have anticoagulant and/ or antiplatelet effects include angelica, bromelain, chamomile, cinnamon, dong quai, evening primrose, feverfew, garlic, ginger, ginkgo biloba, meadowsweet, St John's wort, turmeric and willow bark.

Conversely, some herbal remedies, such as coenzyme Q10 and goldenseal, increase the risk of clotting, a factor that may be significant in the perinatal period when maternal clotting factors naturally increase to prevent torrential haemorrhage at delivery. Theoretically, unreported self-administration of these herbs, particularly over a prolonged period, could significantly disrupt the coagulation mechanism, increasing the risk of disseminated intravascular coagulation in the event of severe postpartum haemorrhage.

Carcinogenicity tends to occur with prolonged use and may not become apparent for some time. Several herbs have been shown to have potential cancer-causing effects, including aloe vera leaf (Guo and Mei 2016). Another herbal remedy, Aristolochia clematitis, also known as birthwort, is used in Chinese medicine, but it is banned in many countries as there is considerable evidence to indicate that it may cause carcinoma in the upper renal tract (Hoang *et al.* 2016).

Musculoskeletal adverse effects tend to be non-specific and may result from toxicity to other systems. Muscle and joint pain may occur, but ataxia, reduced bone density and other symptoms can develop with prolonged exposure to the culpable plants.

Immune system effects can be considerable from herbal remedies and most of the literature explores the immunostimulant action of different plant substances, notably echinacea (Bone 2012; Karsch-Völk *et al.* 2014). However, caution should be employed in women with existing immune system disorders such as rheumatoid arthritis, systemic lupus erythematosus, inflammatory bowel disease, multiple sclerosis, type 1 diabetes mellitus, Guillain-Barre syndrome and psoriasis.

Interactions between NRs and drugs or other herbs

Interactions can occur between herbal remedies and drugs or between two or more herbs used concomitantly. Since herbal remedies, like drugs, are metabolized by the liver, the potential for hepatotoxicity is substantial if NRs are taken injudiciously. Complex cytochrome P450 (CYP450) enzymes (proteins), located in most organs and tissues of the body, act to metabolize endogenous substances in the liver, kidney, lungs, digestive tract and other tissues; this is thought to be the prominent mechanism for processing foreign molecules entering the body. The composition of the CYP450 mechanism is affected by genetic, environmental and lifestyle factors, influencing the metabolism of drugs and other substances. This means that two competing chemicals requiring metabolism by the same CYP450 enzyme may interact with one another, leading to the dominance of one substance over the other (potentiation or prolonged effects), or conversely inhibition (suppressing one substance and increasing the half-life of the other).

Interaction may prevent the full detoxification process of the foreign chemicals or cause retention of metabolites that should have been eliminated, the latter in some cases having a longer-term effect in the form of carcinogenesis. Further, when humans or animals ingest secondary plant metabolites, there can be significant disruption of metabolic pathways within the body, triggering serious adverse effects. St John's wort is a particular example of a popular herbal remedy found to have a significant impact on the CYP450 mechanism in humans; it is known to interact with the contraceptive Pill, anticoagulants, antidepressants, certain antivirals, immunosuppressants, narcotics, digoxin, antirejection drugs used after organ transplant and others (Awortwe *et al.* 2018; Mayo Clinic 2017). On the other hand, some phytochemicals can increase detoxification by inducing CYP450 metabolism, including chemicals found in citrus fruits, particularly grapefruit, plants from the cabbage family, grapes and several spices. Patients on certain drugs are advised to avoid these foods to prevent an overly rapid metabolism.

Common herbal interactions can occur when a woman is taking anticoagulants or antiplatelet medications, including heparin, warfarin and enoxaparin, as well as non-steroidal anti-inflammatories, for example aspirin, particularly in conjunction with therapeutic doses of remedies such as ginger, feverfew or ginkgo biloba and others (Di Minno *et al.* 2017). Antidepressants, notably tricyclics, and monoamine oxidase inhibitors may interact with ginseng, kava and St John's wort (Nicolussi *et al.* 2020), and anti-epilepsy medication may be affected by grapefruit, echinacea, St John's wort and evening primrose (Rašković *et al.* 2014). Nutmeg, either in therapeutic oral doses or inhaled as an essential oil, is hallucinogenic and may interfere with the pharmacology of pethidine (Swerts *et al.* 2014).

Hypoglycaemic effects can occur with some herbs and women with diabetes mellitus should avoid these, although non-diabetics can also experience the effects of a fall in serum glucose. Examples include aloe vera, astralgus, cassia, coenzyme Q10, garlic, ginger, Panax ginseng, Siberian ginseng and St John's wort. Medication for cardiac and cardiovascular conditions may interact with ginger, motherwort, ginseng, liquorice, black pepper essential oil, peppermint essential oil, passiflora, coenzyme Q10 and St John's wort. Kava and coenzyme Q10 are contraindicated with certain antiemetics, whilst other herbs interact with certain anaesthetics, antihistamines, antihypertensives and antacids. Phyoestrogenic herbs such as blue cohosh, ginseng, liquorice, raspberry leaf, red clover, St John's wort and vitex agnus castus should be avoided with oxytocics in labour and postnatally when recommencing the contraceptive Pill.

Pregnancy and labour already place physiological demands on the woman's body, and those who require prescribed medication for obstetric complications or pre-existing medical conditions must be strongly advised to avoid all herbal remedies unless prescribed by a qualified, experienced medical herbalist. Caution is needed when using aromatherapy essential oils and TMs to avoid either complicating the symptom picture further or masking any worsening of the mother's condition.

Specific adverse effects of NRs on pregnancy and labour

A comprehensive systematic review of almost a hundred studies involving over a million pregnant women showed significant negative effects from inappropriate use of herbal remedies (Muñoz Balbontín *et al.* 2019). For example, raspberry leaf was shown to be associated with an increased need for Caesarean section; liquorice and ingestion of sweet almond oil were associated with preterm labour; and several studies found evidence of interactions between herbal remedies and obstetric drugs (Brantley *et al.* 2014; Illamola *et al.* 2020; Lake and Olana Fite 2019). Amongst the indigenous African population, antenatal and intrapartum use of NRs is associated with a high rate of postnatal and neonatal complications (Fukunaga *et al.* 2020). Increasingly, expectant mothers are putting their own and their unborn babies' health at risk due to lack of knowledge about NRs, notably herbal medicines and aromatherapy essential oils, as well as a general lack of communication with their healthcare providers who are, in turn, poorly informed (Bruno *et al.* 2018).

There are many herbal remedies and TMs that are completely contraindicated in the preconception period, pregnancy, labour and during breastfeeding. Examples include, but are not restricted to:

- Aconite
- Agrimony
- Ashwagandha
- Belladonna
- Birthwort
- Blue cohosh
- Boldo
- Butterbur
- Cascarilla

- Cinchona
- Colchicum
- Coltsfoot
- Comfrey
- Deadly nightshade
- Henbane
- Kava
- Khat
- Lady's mantle

- Lobelia
- Opium
- Pennyroyal
- Rue
- Staphysagria
- Tansy
- Wormseed
- Wormwood
- Yohimbe

When NRs are used in the preconception period and early pregnancy, there are risks of teratogenicity and mutagenicity. For example, Lin *et al.* (2019) found an association of ginseng and other Chinese herbs with low birth weight and preterm birth when taken by women undergoing assisted reproduction. Many herbal remedies cross the placenta and may be toxic to the embryo, including autumn crocus, comfrey, mistletoe, pennyroyal, pokeroot, tansy and wormwood and herbs used in Chinese medicine (Li *et al.* 2015). Even the ubiquitous ginger, an extremely popular remedy for pregnancy sickness, may be teratogenic in large quantities and contribute to fetal loss (Eid and Jaradat 2020; Stanisiere, Mousset and Lafay 2018). Others are known abortifacients (causing uterine contractions) or emmenagoguic (causing menstruation-like vaginal bleeding) and can, on occasion, be fatal (Ossei *et al.* 2020). Emmenagoguic NRs increase the risk of threatened miscarriage, antepartum or postpartum haemorrhage, whilst those that trigger contractions may contribute to preterm labour, intrapartum hypertonic uterine activity or excessive postnatal bleeding in susceptible women.

Some NRs may also have adverse effects on neonates, especially with prolonged use during pregnancy or excessive use near term. For example, cannabis may contribute to an increased risk of psychotic-like episodes in neonates (Bolhuis *et al.* 2018; Gunn *et al.* 2016), and there have been several reports over the years of serious neonatal effects of blue cohosh, commonly used in the USA to expedite labour, including epileptic-type convulsions, stroke and congestive heart failure (Datta *et al.* 2014; Dugoua *et al.* 2008; Finkel and Zarlengo 2004; MacPherson and Kilminster 2006).

Essential oils work somewhat differently in respect of embryological risk. Although essential oil molecules cross the placental barrier, the risk of toxicity depends on the concentration, method of administration (respiratory or dermal) and the proportion of different chemicals thought to have adverse effects on cell formation. Conversely, essential oils known to have emmenagoguic properties may contribute to threatened or actual miscarriage. However, it is fair to state that when used appropriately in minimal doses up to a maximum of 1.5 per cent, some – but certainly not all – essential oils should be "safe enough" in pregnancy. Women should be advised to avoid all aromatherapy oils unless they are informed that they are safe to use. Most issues with essential oil safety arise from a desire to enjoy the aromatic benefits without understanding the pharmacological impact of aromatherapy.

Self-administration of herbal remedies and TMs in conjunction with drugs prescribed for a specific clinical indication is of concern, not least due to non-disclosure. A common example is the use of NRs such as raspberry leaf or clary sage essential oil to encourage uterine contractions at the same time as oxytocic induction of labour is undertaken (source: numerous communications with colleagues). Until further evidence is available on the safety of NRs for induction of labour, it is recommended that they are not used (Zamawe *et al.* 2018). It is essential that women are questioned about their use of NRs immediately prior to and during labour, even when it is of spontaneous onset. Continuation of intrapartum self-administration of uterotonic herbs can lead to disturbed uterine polarity, hypertonic or hypotonic contractions, fetal distress and, in extreme circumstances, placental separation and catastrophic haemorrhage or uterine rupture with fetal and maternal death.

Herbs and oils contraindicated in pregnancy due to their potential to cause uterine contractions include:

• Angelica	• Clary sage	• Mugwort
• Aniseed	• Clove bud	• Oregano
• Arbor vitae	• Cowslip	• Parsley
• Ashwagandha	• Devil's claw	• Passiflora
• Barberry	• Dong quai	• Raspberry leaf
• Basil	• False unicorn root	• Rosemary
• Betony	• Fennel	• Saffron
• Bitter orange	• Fenugreek	• Sage
• Black cohosh	• Ginger	• Shepherd's purse
• Bloodroot	• Goldenseal	• Thyme
• Blue cohosh	• Jasmine	• Turmeric
• Caraway	• Juniper berry	• Vervain
• Celery seed	• Marjoram	• Wild yam
• Cinnamon	• Motherwort	• Yarrow

(Note: Small amounts of those herbs commonly used in cooking are generally safe and some are suitable for use with caution during or after labour.)

Altered physiology during the childbearing year further increases the risks from metabolism of NRs. For example, glomerular filtration fluctuations impact on renal excretion of chemical substances, and glucose metabolism may be impaired when NRs with hypoglycaemic potential are used, such as ginseng, fenugreek and bitter melon, as well as various plants used in Chinese and Ayurvedic medicine (Hui, Tang and Go 2009). Similarly, the natural haemodilution in pregnancy may be exacerbated by herbs known to reduce iron levels, such as turmeric, possibly leading to pathological anaemia (Smith and Ashar 2019).

Contraindications and precautions to use of NRs in pregnancy and childbirth

It is fascinating to note, in the debate on the safe use of NRs, that very few authorities apply the principles of NR risk to the complexities of specific medical conditions. There is a dichotomy between orthodox and complementary medical advice. The conventional healthcare sector usually states generic contraindications, primarily in relation to herbal medicines, as: pregnancy and breastfeeding; concomitant use with prescribed drugs; serious health issues such as liver or kidney disease; impending elective surgery; and children under 18 and adults over 65 years of age. This broad advice is wise but is not specific enough, is not based on any in-depth professional knowledge of doctors and pharmacists, and fails to take account of the increasing self-administration of herbal remedies by the general public. The added injunction to "contact your doctor or pharmacist before taking herbal remedies" is also not particularly helpful, especially since some medical practitioners disparage NRs, and many will not have adequate knowledge of the pertinent issues of self-administering NRs; thus the potential that patients will not seek guidance is very real.

Similarly, conventional healthcare sources state, correctly, that homeopathic remedies may contain potentially harmful substances yet fail to set this in the context of the mechanism of action of homeopathy, by which the toxicity of substances prepared homeopathically (that is, diluted and succussed) is rendered pharmacologically inactive. An example is the use of arsenic. Many people are aware that arsenic can be fatal in large doses and may cause profuse vomiting, diarrhoea, headache, tachycardia and palpitations in lower doses – these are adverse reactions to the chemicals. However, homeopathic arsenic treats the same symptom picture, with any changes in symptoms being healing aggravations rather than the toxic effects of arsenic.

European, US and Australian government attitudes towards TMs and "folk medicine" from China, India, Africa and elsewhere is similarly judgemental, implying an intrinsic belief that, since TMs originate from cultural groups, largely in developing countries, they cannot possibly be as safe, reliable, effective or acceptable as conventional pharmaceutical drugs. The pharmaceutical companies come under extensive criticism in this respect, although in fairness, many companies are investigating the components of TMs for development into mainstream drugs. The arrogant attitudes of western governments towards TMs may only partly be attributed to the commercialization of the pharmaceutical industry; the real issues go beyond this to an inherent distrust of anything that is not home grown and that does not fit contemporary established principles.

On the other hand, in regions of the world where TMs are used by large numbers of the indigenous populations, government approval may take a different stance. For example, in Africa, whilst TMs are not necessarily incorporated into allopathic medicine, a greater appreciation of the public's reliance on TMs has led many governments to develop national policies and regulatory frameworks for TM. By 2010, 22 African countries were engaged in research on the medicinal potential of plants used in TM, and the number of marketing authorizations for individual TM products ranged from 1 in Cameroon to over 1000 in Ghana and Nigeria; several countries also included TMs in their lists of nationally approved drugs (Mothibe and Sibanda 2019). The Japanese government tacitly acknowledges the place of kampo, and China and India are making rapid progress in integrating TMs further into conventional healthcare. However, in the Far East, since national personality characteristics favour deference to authority, governmental advice focuses more on seeking help from appropriately trained practitioners of TM rather than on the issues of self-administration, despite the increasing availability of over-the-counter remedies.

Generic government-produced safety statements in westernized countries are intended to cover the widest range of the general public and serve to relinquish any real sense of responsibility since herbal, homeopathic and traditional remedies are not generally part of a country's orthodox healthcare system. The popular media reinforces this by sensationalizing case studies in which people have suffered severe, often fatal or bizarre adverse effects, using disparaging and inflammatory language, and generally siding with the prevailing government advice. Conversely, sources of public information from complementary medical organizations tend to focus on the benefits of remedies prescribed by trained practitioners or those that can be self-prescribed and administered. Essentially, conventional healthcare authorities focus on the potential negative effects of NRs whilst complementary medicine organizations focus on the positive side as an alternative to pharmaceutical preparations.

All of this is sensible, if slightly ambiguous, advice, on both sides of the dilemma, but it does not take account of the tsunami of ill-informed self-administration of NRs, particularly when combined with conventional healthcare. Nowhere is this more significant than in maternity care. There are some women in whom NRs should be avoided completely (see above), whilst for others there will be some precautions, based on their individual medical or obstetric history and current condition. Despite this, Kennedy *et al.*'s comprehensive survey (2013) identified 126 specific herbal medicines being used by pregnant women, of which 27 were contraindicated at this time and 60 were classified as "requiring caution in pregnancy".

As a basic rule of thumb, women in the preconception, antenatal, intrapartum and postnatal periods, whose medical and obstetric conditions fit into the spectrum of physiological normality, may be eligible to use certain NRs if they so choose, subject to the issues previously discussed in respect of appropriate selection and doses, recognition of adverse reactions and avoidance of any remedies contraindicated at this time. For all other women, it is necessary to determine those for whom NR use is an absolute contraindication and those in whom caution may be required. In reality, this can be difficult and tends to be a matter of degree. It may be related to the specific condition and its severity, such as whether it is acute or chronic, obstetric-related or a general medical condition. Safety may depend on the specific NR the woman intends to use and whether it is prescribed by a suitably qualified practitioner or is self-administered. The modality of the NR may dictate whether or not it is safe in any given situation, for example herbal or homeopathic medicines.

Any woman with maternal, fetal or general obstetric pathology, especially those requiring medical intervention or pharmaceutical drugs, should avoid all NRs. Those with pre-existing medical conditions or incidental non-obstetric-related pathology developing during pregnancy should also avoid using NRs. The interaction between the disease process and the normal physiological adaptations of pregnancy place an already heavy burden on the woman's system, which the use of NRs can only complicate further. Major pre-existing hepatic, renal, cardiac and neurological conditions, as well as women living with cancer, fall into this category (Damery *et al.* 2011). Indeed, any woman requiring hospitalization during pregnancy for any reason other than physiological labour must be asked if she is taking any NRs and be strongly advised to stop. She should be advised that continuing to do so may compromise her condition and may affect the medical treatment she is able to receive. Should a woman decide to continue her use of NRs, medical staff, including obstetricians, paediatricians, anaesthetists and other attending physicians, must be advised, and the fact of her self-administration highlighted in the medical notes. Similarly, maternity carers providing NRs such as essential oils in the form of aromatherapy should discontinue their use in the event of pathological complications developing.

Table 3 identifies some of the medical and obstetric contraindications and precautions to the use of NRs. A few major medical or obstetric conditions are considered absolute contraindications; all others are precautions to the use of NRs and healthcare professionals should employ all normal judicious decision-making to determine the appropriateness or otherwise of NR use for individual use.

Table 3: Contraindications and precautions to NRs

System	General medical conditions	Pregnancy-induced conditions
Hepato-biliary/ renal systems	Severe renal disease*	Obstetric cholestasis*
	Liver disease, cirrhosis, transplant*	Acute fatty liver of pregnancy*
		HELLP syndrome*
	High intake of substances metabolized by liver including recreational drugs, alcohol dependence*	Recurrent urinary tract infections
	Gall bladder disease, gall stones, renal calculi	
Cardiovascular/ haematological systems	Anticoagulants, antiplatelet drugs*	Prophylactic aspirin, heparin, warfarin, enoxaparin, etc.
	Coagulation disorders, e.g. von Willebrand's disease, thrombocytopaenia, haemophilia, antiphospholipid syndrome	Threatened miscarriage, antepartum haemorrhage
		Severe primary or secondary postpartum haemorrhage
		Symptomatic uterine fibroids
	History of embolism, DVT, severe thrombophlebitis*	Deep vein thrombosis, pulmonary embolism*
	Essential hypertension	Disseminated intravascular dissemination due to major postpartum haemorrhage*
	Iron deficiency, sickle cell, other anaemias, folic acid deficiency	Severe varicose veins
		Gestational hypertension, pre-eclampsia
		Pregnancy-induced anaemia, folic acid deficiency

Neurological system	Epilepsy* Migraines, frequent or requiring medication Multiple sclerosis History of stroke	Eclampsia* Guillain-Barre syndrome* Intractable headaches, cluster headaches in pregnancy Bell's palsy or stroke occurring during pregnancy/postnatal period
Gastrointestinal system	Irritable bowel disease, Crohn's disease, diverticulitis, ulcerative colitis, gastric/peptic ulcer Excessive vomiting of unknown cause	Severe oesophageal reflux requiring medication Hyperemesis gravidarum*
Endocrine system	Diabetes mellitus Thyroid disease Cushing syndrome, Addison's disease Pituitary tumours	Gestational diabetes Gestational thyroid conditions Molar pregnancy, chorioncarcinoma, phaeochromocytoma Postpartum hypopituitarism
Respiratory/ pulmonary system	Asthma Pneumonia, tuberculosis	Dyspnoea – consider differential diagnosis, e.g. gestational anaemia
Immune system	Major infections of any type or origin; pyrexia Tendency to/history of allergic reactions Cancers of any type or origin Systemic lupus erythematosus Antiphospholipid syndrome HIV/AIDS	Major infections of any type or origin; pyrexia Autoimmune conditions precipitated by pregnancy*
Integumentary/ musculoskeletal systems	Skin sensitivities, severe eczema, psoriasis Any musculoskeletal condition requiring regular medication, particularly if metabolized via the liver	Obstetric cholestasis*
Psycho-social issues	Schizophrenia, bipolar syndrome* Substance misuse/dependency* Morbid obesity	Antenatal/postnatal depression requiring medication*

System	General medical conditions	Pregnancy-induced conditions
Reproductive system	Uterine fibroids, endometriosis Fertility issues – notably assisted reproduction Hormone-sensitive cancers – breast, ovary, uterus, cervix* Sexually transmitted infections Polycystic ovarian syndrome	Maternal obstetric complications, identified by systems above Preterm labour, history of precipitate labour Multiple pregnancy, especially higher multiples Abnormal presentation/lie – breech, transverse, unstable, etc. Placental insufficiency, fetal growth retardation or macrosomia History of repeated fetal loss, i.e. miscarriage, stillbirth Fetal abnormalities Booked for elective Caesarean section*

Note: * = Absolute contraindication.

It is essential that maternity carers are able to differentiate between a normal healing reaction, a reverse proving, an adverse reaction to a therapeutic dose or a side effect of inappropriate administration or overdose. In reality, it can be difficult to differentiate between a reaction to a normal therapeutic dose of a remedy and adverse effects caused by overdose. Furthermore, maternity professionals must distinguish between NR-related reactions and the normal physiological effects of pregnancy or emerging pathology. For example, if a woman has used a remedy and then develops a headache, this could be due to tiredness, stress or dehydration, it may be a direct or indirect reaction to the remedy, or it could herald worsening pre-eclampsia. Skin irritation may be a normal healing reaction to an NR, an adverse reaction, a side effect of inappropriate administration, physiological pruritis or developing pathology such as cholestasis. It is paramount that pregnant women are asked about their use of NRs, since any true adverse reactions may be missed or misinterpreted and a diagnosis of toxicity may therefore be delayed. There is also a need for vigilance when women self-administer TMs from their own cultures with which midwives and obstetricians are almost certainly unfamiliar, even when TMs are integrated into family life (Singh and Zhao 2017).

It is also possible that true adverse effects of NRs in pregnancy and childbirth are seriously under-reported, both through lack of knowledge of individual remedies and ignorance of women's self-administration (Walji *et al.* 2009). In the UK, adverse drug reactions, side effects and interactions are reported to the Medicines & Healthcare products Regulatory Authority using the Yellow Card system; the same mechanism can be used to report adverse reactions to herbal, homeopathic and traditional remedies. Plant adverse reactions can also be reported to the Poisons Unit at Guy's Hospital in London, which works in conjunction with Kew Gardens to document all reports. Similar reporting systems are in use in the USA (via the MedWatch system of the FDA), Canada (MedEffect), the EU (European Medicines Agency), Australia (Therapeutic Goods Administration), South Africa (SA Health Products Regulatory Authority) and in most other countries.

Added to the pharmacological effects of NRs are the human factors that influence women's use of NRs. Pregnant women's desires to avoid prescribed drugs, to use "natural" rather than manufactured substances, to expedite the birth and to retain control over the childbearing process may contribute unwittingly to a more serious situation requiring medical intervention and, in labour, possible transfer from home or a low-risk birth centre to an obstetric unit. The ready availability of information sources (whether correct or incorrect, both by inclusion or omission) and of over-the-counter remedies multiplies the risks of using NRs in pregnancy, labour or the postnatal period.

Healthcare providers working with pregnant, labouring and newly birthed mothers must be able to assess women who choose to self-administer NRs or who seek professional advice outside the conventional maternity services. Maternity professionals who integrate NRs such as aromatherapy or homeopathy into their practice must be conscious of the individual clinical implications as well as the local, regional, national and international regulations pertaining to NR use and work within the legal parameters of their own professions. Midwives and doctors must also be vigilant to the potential for interactions of NRs with any medication the mother may require.

4

Guidelines for Healthcare Professionals

General notes

- The definition of "natural remedies" (NRs) includes all herbal remedies, herbal teas, aromatherapy essential oils, homeopathic medicines, tissue salts and flower remedies, plus traditional (indigenous) medicines, whether sourced from plants, minerals or animals.

- All NRs should be treated with the same respect as that given to pharmaceutical drugs. It is essential to differentiate between herbal and homeopathic/energy-based remedies – the Latin name may be the same, but safety concerns differ depending on the mechanism of action.

- NRs may be prescribed by appropriately qualified independent practitioners, self-administered by pregnant women from over-the-counter remedies, or integrated into conventional maternity care by midwives, doctors and doulas. They may be taken orally, applied to the skin, inhaled or prescribed by qualified NR practitioners for administration *per rectum*, *per vaginam* or, rarely, by intravenous or subcutaneous injection.

- "Natural" does not mean that all NRs are safe, or safe for all, particularly during pregnancy and childbirth. No NR should be used routinely for prolonged periods of time. Natural remedies should not be used as a replacement for proven medical treatment, especially in the event of an emergency.

Gaining information about NRs from pregnant, labouring or breastfeeding women

- It is wise to assume that a large proportion of women using the maternity services may be self-administering NRs and that some will decline to reveal their use, even when questioned.

- Women should be advised to avoid ALL NRs before and during pregnancy, labour and breastfeeding unless under the supervision of an appropriately qualified, insured professional.

- Women should be asked at their first antenatal appointment if they are using any NRs and their answers recorded in the maternity notes. It may be necessary to be explicit about the definition of "natural remedies" to encompass the wide spectrum of modalities. Women should be asked again about their use of NRs in the third trimester as they prepare for the birth, and in early labour, to ascertain if they are using any remedies that may compromise maternal or fetal wellbeing or progress. In labour, any NR use should be documented in the labour record and correlated with any technological monitoring systems (such as a cardiotocograph). Lactating mothers should also be asked about their use of NRs.

- Practitioners of herbal, homeopathic or other traditional medicines and complementary therapies, as well as pharmacists and point-of-sales staff in natural health stores, should ask women seeking NRs if they are, or could be, pregnant, are breastfeeding or undergoing fertility treatment.

Advice to women taking NRs

- Women should be advised to seek professional advice on NRs and not to rely on information obtained from the internet, social and other media or friends and family. Women should avoid using NRs given to them by non-professionals – what one woman uses may not be appropriate or safe for another.

- Women should be informed that not all NRs are approved, regulated or evidence-based. NRs obtained from the internet may be falsely labelled, contaminated with chemical impurities or contain banned or toxic ingredients.

- Women should be informed about the possible risks of taking pharmacologically active NRs, including adverse effects such as allergies and interactions with other NRs, prescribed medications or foods. They should also be helped to understand healing reactions and reverse provings caused by energetic medicines such as homeopathy. They should be advised to report any untoward symptoms to their maternity carers and, if relevant, to their independent NR practitioners.

- If a woman reveals her use of NRs, the precise remedies must be identified (by Latin names where possible) and recorded. She should be advised to commence with the lowest dose and not to exceed the recommended maximum dose.

- Advise women against combining several different NRs/complementary therapies: take only one remedy at a time, particularly at term, when women may seek to expedite labour.

Specific information on using essential oils in aromatherapy

- Women should generally be advised to avoid all essential oils during pregnancy unless professionally prescribed. If they disclose their self-use of essential oils, this should be documented.

- Women should be advised to purchase good quality essential oils; they must be stored in a refrigerator and discarded after the expiry date or if the aroma changes (which may be a sign of chemical deterioration). They should be advised to use essential oil doses of no more than 1.5 per cent in pregnancy and 2 per cent in labour and postnatally.

- Essential oils should not be applied to the skin neat; they should not be taken orally, rectally or used in or around the vaginal opening; keep them away from eyes.

- Essential oils should not be used in the birthing pool in labour, or in the bath once the membranes have ruptured, and should be discontinued once the second stage commences to avoid exposing the newborn baby to the vapours (chemicals).

- Aromatherapy should not be used concomitantly with homeopathic remedies that may be antidoted by the strong aromas.

- It is unsafe to use diffusers/vaporizers in an institutional setting such as a maternity unit or birth centre, particularly in public areas where mothers, staff and visitors may inhale chemicals that are unsafe or that may trigger adverse reactions. Aromatherapy diffusers in the home should be used for no more than 15 minutes in any hour; do not use near babies, children, older people or animals. Maternity professionals attending women at home in labour who choose to use diffusers should be alert to the adverse effects on themselves which may arise from inhalation of specific chemicals from the oils.

- Pregnant maternity professionals must avoid working with women using oils intended to promote uterine contractions during labour, for example clary sage and jasmine. Birth companions who may be pregnant should also not be exposed to vapours from uterine-contracting oils.

- Caution should also be employed to ensure individuals in contact with the chemical vapours do not have major medical conditions or allergies that could be adversely affected by inhalation of the essential oil chemicals.

- Newborn babies should not be exposed to essential oil aromas during the birth, when breastfeeding or in the room where they sleep; *never* use essential oils directly on, or for, babies.

Women who choose to continue using NRs against professional advice

- Unless under the supervision of a qualified NR practitioner, women should be encouraged to stop or reduce their use of NRs. Discontinuation may need to be gradual to reduce the risks of sudden withdrawal.

- Women who continue using NRs against medical advice should be advised to leave two hours between administration of the NRs and any prescribed medications; their decision to continue should be documented in their maternity notes.

- Women with any medical, obstetric or fetal pathology, either pre-existing, gestationally induced or occurring incidentally during pregnancy, labour or the early postnatal period, should be advised to avoid self-medication of all NRs.

- NRs are completely contraindicated for pregnant women with major hepatic, renal, cardiac and neurological conditions and cancers of any type, irrespective of whether they currently require pharmaceutical medications. Those taking medically prescribed drugs, by whatever route of administration, should be strongly advised against using NRs at any time.

- Maternity professionals should be alert to the possibility that deviations from normal progress in pregnancy or labour may be linked with undisclosed use of NRs and should question women about their possible use of NRs. It is vital that maternity professionals can identify women's symptoms and differentiate between adverse reactions to NRs, normal obstetric physiology or emerging pathological complications, and recognize interactions between NRs and drugs.

- Women admitted to the antenatal ward have, by definition, pathological complications requiring medical attention; they must be asked directly if they are self-administering NRs. It is not appropriate for midwives and other maternity professionals to advocate NRs for these women or to use essential oils for aromatherapy in the antenatal ward area.

- Women should be advised to discontinue all pharmacologically active NRs (herbal and traditional medicines) at least two weeks prior to elective surgery or dental extraction to reduce the risk of excessive bleeding. Anaesthetists and dental surgeons should check whether women have continued to use NRs immediately prior to surgery, some of which may have an adverse effect on blood clotting.

Interprofessional communication

- Conventional maternity records should routinely incorporate a question on women's use of NRs, in the antenatal history and labour records, to ensure all care providers are aware of the potential for adverse effects and interactions with drugs. Maternity professionals should encourage women seeking independent NR advice to inform pharmacists, NR practitioners or point-of-sales staff in natural health stores that they are pregnant or breastfeeding.

- Independent practitioners of complementary therapies who incorporate NRs into their treatment of, or advice to, clients should encourage women to inform their conventional maternity carers or take steps to interact directly with obstetricians and midwives when working with pregnant clients.

- In the event of obstetric complications or exacerbation of pre-existing medical conditions requiring the transfer of a woman from home or a low-risk centre to a high-risk medical facility, maternity professionals must inform those taking over the care if the woman has received or been self-administering any NRs. This is particularly significant in labour.

- Midwives, doctors and doulas and other conventional healthcare professionals working with pregnant women should consult qualified practitioners of the relevant NR modality for more in-depth information, especially in the event of clinical issues arising which may be related to women's NR use.

- Healthcare professionals from all disciplines, whether conventional or complementary, should be encouraged to report any suspected adverse reactions to the relevant national medicines or healthcare products regulatory authority.

Professional education and research

- All relevant healthcare professionals should acquire a basic knowledge of how the metabolism of NRs can affect pregnancy and childbirth and *vice versa*, and particularly how to differentiate between normal physiology, adverse reactions to NRs and emerging obstetric pathology.

- Medical, midwifery and health visitor pre-registration education and doula and antenatal teacher preparation should include an appropriate introduction to the safe use of NRs in pregnancy and childbirth that balances benefits and risks.

- Complementary therapy practitioner education should include a mandatory module, either at pre-registration or post-registration level, on the application of the specific NR modality or complementary therapy to pregnancy and breastfeeding.

- There is an urgent need for more research on the safety of NRs, not simply their effectiveness. Not all NR modalities can be studied using a randomized, controlled, blinded approach. Healthcare professionals engaged in research projects investigating the effectiveness of NRs should ensure their knowledge of the NR modality is sufficient to ensure the safety of subjects in the trial.

5

Alphabetical Listing of Natural Remedies

ACACIA

Acacia senegal, Acacia arabica Herbal remedy, also known as Arabic gum.

Indications: Orally – for irritable bowel syndrome, hypercholesterolaemia, diabetes mellitus, obesity, for detoxification, a healthy gut. Topically – for dental plaque, gingivitis, skin inflammation.

Safety in pregnancy: Appears safe in amounts commonly used in foods and in therapeutic doses in the short term.

Contraindications and precautions: Avoid with asthma or allergy to rye grass and other grass pollens. Caution in diabetes mellitus: may affect serum glucose levels.

Adverse effects: Abdominal bloating, nausea, diarrhoea; hypoglycaemia.

Interactions: Therapeutic oral doses, prolonged, excessive or inappropriate use may interact with amoxycillin, antidiabetic medication. Hypoglycaemic herbs: cassia cinnamon, devil's claw, guar gum, Panax ginseng, Siberian ginseng.

ACAI BERRY

Euterpe oleracea Herbal remedy.

Indications: Orally – for constipation, gut health, weight loss, general health and wellbeing; as a nutritional supplement.

Safety in pregnancy: Appears safe in amounts commonly used in foods. Caution: insufficient information on safety of therapeutic doses in pregnancy.

Contraindications and precautions: Allergy to berry fruits; pre-existing or gestational diabetes; hypotension. Do not confuse with Acacia.

Adverse effects: May affect blood pressure and blood sugar levels. Raw fruit/juice may be contaminated with protozoa.

Interactions: No drug or herb interactions documented, but in view of potential adverse effects, the advice is to avoid therapeutic oral doses, prolonged, excessive or inappropriate use with antidiabetic medication and antihypertensives, and with hypoglycaemic and hypotensive herbs: aloe vera, berberine, cassia cinnamon, devil's claw, guar gum, Panax ginseng, Siberian ginseng.

ACONITE
Aconitum napellus, Aconitum carmichaeli Herbal remedy, also known as Monk's hood.

Indications: Orally – for irregular menstruation. Also for joint pain, gastroenteritis, diarrhoea, asthma, inflammation, skin diseases, to induce sweating. Topically – for facial neuralgia, skin inflammation, sciatica. Used in Chinese, Korean and Indian Ayurvedic medicine.

Safety in pregnancy: AVOID IN PREGNANCY, LABOUR AND BREASTFEEDING – the root contains fast-acting toxic alkaloids that affect the heart and central nervous system.

Contraindications and precautions: Some other herbal products can occasionally be contaminated with aconite, causing adverse effects similar to aconite toxicity. Do not confuse with homeopathic Aconite.

Adverse effects: Nausea, vomiting, dilated pupils, muscle weakness, hypotension, hypoglycaemia, hypokalaemia, acidosis, neurological effects, bradycardia or tachycardia; pulmonary oedema, loss of consciousness, death.

Interactions: Minimal oral or topical amounts may interact with anticoagulants and antiplatelet drugs: heparin, warfarin, aspirin, diclofenac, ibuprofen, enoxaparin; may also interact with stimulant drugs. Anticoagulant herbs: angelica, clove, garlic, ginger, ginkgo, meadowsweet, Panax ginseng, poplar, red clover, turmeric. Stimulating herbs: angelica, basil, camphor, coffee, kola nut, nutmeg, rosemary, tansy, wintergreen, yerba mate.

ACONITE
Aconitum napellus Homeopathic remedy, from Monk's hood.

Obstetric indications: Labour – late, with fear of going into labour. Contractions violent, severe, rapid, relentless and ineffective; soreness in the lower back; fetal malposition; pain – intolerable, intense, tearing, like knives. Shock after Caesarean or fast labour.

Key features: Sudden onset of symptoms due to trauma, shock, fright or exposure to cold, dry conditions; restlessness; localized part may feel contracted; thirsty for bitter drinks; bitter taste in mouth; sweat on uncovered parts; tachycardia, hypertension.

Emotional symptoms: Panic, terror, acute anxiety; fear impending death (mother and baby).

Better for: Open air; rest; lying down.

Worse for: Stuffy environment; noise and music; feeling chilled; emotional outbursts.

Safety: Primarily used for acute, sudden onset conditions; should not normally be used for chronic conditions unless under the supervision of a qualified homeopath. Do not use if there are any medical or obstetric complications. Not to be used as a replacement for standard medical care. Do not use with aromatherapy essential oils, topically or by inhalation, or with antacids, decongestants, laxatives or cough lozenges – inactivates the remedy. Do not take with food or drink. Do not take prophylactically – may lead to reverse proving. Should not be used by women who do not fit the symptom picture to avoid reverse proving. To be handled by the intended recipient only. Do not confuse with Aconite, the herbal remedy.

AFRICAN COFFEE TREE *see* Cascara

AFRICAN GERANIUM *see* Umckaloabo

AFRICAN MARIGOLD *see* Marigold

AGRIMONY
Agrimonia eupatoria Herbal remedy.

Indications: Orally – as a diuretic; for a sore throat; diarrhoea or irritable bowel syndrome; as a sedative, antihistamine, anti-inflammatory, antibacterial, antiviral; diabetes mellitus, gallbladder disorders. Topically – as a mild astringent; for skin inflammation; as a gargle for sore throats. Also available as liquid Bach Flower Rescue Remedy taken orally, diluted in spring water, for doubt and a negative outlook.

Safety in pregnancy: AVOID ORAL USE IN PREGNANCY, LABOUR AND BREASTFEEDING – possible hormonal activity could lead to miscarriage, preterm labour. Bach Flower Rescue Remedy appears safe.

Contraindications and precautions: Do not confuse with Agrimony, the homeopathic remedy. Do not confuse with hemp agrimony. Avoid Bach Flower Rescue Remedy with liver disease, alcohol dependency, severe mental health issues.

Adverse effects: Diarrhoea, nausea, vomiting or constipation due to tannin content. Anaemia due to poor iron absorption as a result of high tannin levels. Bruising, bleeding and possible kidney damage with long-term use.

Interactions: Therapeutic oral doses, prolonged, excessive or inappropriate use may interact with antidiabetic medication. Absorption of any medication taken orally may be inhibited due to high tannin levels. Hypoglycaemic herbs: cassia cinnamon, devil's claw, guar gum, Panax ginseng, Siberian ginseng.

ALCHEMILLA *see* Lady's mantle

ALFALFA
Medicago sativa Herbal remedy, also known as Lucerne.

Indications: Orally – for menopausal symptoms. Also as a diuretic, for asthma, arthritis, osteoporosis, diabetes mellitus, as a food supplement.

Safety in pregnancy: Appears safe in amounts commonly used in foods. AVOID THERAPEUTIC DOSES ORALLY IN PRECONCEPTION PERIOD, PREGNANCY AND BREASTFEEDING – contains plant oestrogens, may cause poor implantation, miscarriage, preterm labour and theoretically interfere with lactation.

Contraindications and precautions: Avoid with iron deficiency anaemia and autoimmune diseases.

Adverse effects: Photosensitivity; excessive, prolonged ingestion of seeds may induce lupus effects. Consumption of ground alfalfa seeds may reduce red cells, white cells and platelets in the blood.

Interactions: Therapeutic oral doses, prolonged, excessive or inappropriate use may interact with anticoagulants and antiplatelet drugs: heparin, warfarin, aspirin, diclofenac, ibuprofen, enoxaparin. May also interact with vitamin E, iron, contraceptive Pill, hormone replacement therapy; photosensitizing drugs. Anticoagulant herbs: angelica, clove, garlic, ginger, ginkgo, meadowsweet, Panax ginseng, poplar, red clover, turmeric. Oestrogenic herbs: black cohosh, blue cohosh, dong quai, evening primrose, fennel, fenugreek, ginkgo, ginseng, liquorice, raspberry leaf, red clover, vitex agnus castus.

ALLIUM CEPA
Homeopathic remedy from red onion.

Obstetric indications: Sinus congestion, nasal catarrh, watery eyes; common cold during pregnancy.

Key features: Symptoms similar to those when peeling onions – stinging eyes, burning discharge and a tendency to rub eyes that are red, swollen and itchy. Excessive, watery catarrh, a burning sensation causing excoriation of the upper lip and nostrils. Violent sneezing and cough; constant rhinitis, starting on the left and moving to the right; one-sided nasal congestion.

Emotional symptoms: Fear of pain, general anxiety, melancholy.

Better for: Being in the open air; cold air.

Worse for: Warm rooms; evening; smell of flowers.

Safety: Do not use if there are any medical or obstetric complications. Not to be used as a replacement for standard medical care. Do not use with aromatherapy essential oils, topically or by inhalation, or with antacids, decongestants, laxatives or cough lozenges – inactivates the remedy. Do not take with food or drink. Do not take prophylactically – may lead to reverse proving. Should not be used by women who do not fit the symptom picture to avoid reverse proving. To be handled by the intended recipient only.

ALOE VERA
Aloe vera, Aloe barbadensis Herbal remedy.

Indications: Aloe latex orally – for constipation, weight loss, inflammatory bowel disease, gastroduodenal ulcers. Aloe extract orally – for hyperlipidaemia. Extract and gel topically – for dry skin, seborrheic dermatitis, psoriasis, acne, herpes simplex, nappy rash, scabies, wound healing, striae gravidarum, pressure sores, sunburn, haemorrhoids, dental caries, gingivitis. Aloe leaf juice topically – for anal fissures.

Safety in pregnancy: Topical application generally safe. AVOID ORAL USE OF ALL ALOE PRODUCTS IN PREGNANCY AND BREASTFEEDING – latex and aloe whole leaf extracts also contain anthraquinones that have possible mutagenic and abortifacient effects; may pass to breast milk.

Contraindications and precautions: Avoid oral aloe gel. Caution: some commercial products labelled "aloe juice" may contain whole leaf extract. Do not confuse with Yucca (Aloe yucca).

Adverse effects: Aloe latex orally – abdominal pain, diarrhoea, potassium depletion, proteinuria, muscle weakness, haematuria, gastritis, acute renal failure; may be carcinogenic (conflicting evidence). Topical aloe gel – burning, itching, eczema, contact dermatitis. Aloe leaf extract orally – acute hepatitis.

Interactions: Therapeutic oral doses, prolonged, excessive or inappropriate use may interact with anticoagulants and antiplatelet drugs: heparin, warfarin, aspirin, diclofenac, ibuprofen, enoxaparin. May also interact with antidiabetic medication, diuretics, laxatives, digoxin. Oral aloe latex may interfere with the absorption of any medication taken orally. Anticoagulant herbs: angelica, clove, garlic, ginger, ginkgo, meadowsweet, poplar, red clover, turmeric. Hypoglycaemic herbs: cassia, cinnamon, devil's claw, Panax ginseng, Siberian ginseng. Also horsetail and liquorice, which may interfere with potassium levels.

ALOE YUCCA *see* Yucca

AMERICAN CONE FLOWER *see* Echinacea

AMERICAN VALERIAN *see* **Nerve root**

ANGELICA
Angelica archangelica/officinalis Herbal remedy, also known as Danggui.

Indications: Orally – to induce menstrual flow, as an abortifacient. Also for indigestion, flatulence, loss of appetite; as a diuretic; antiseptic, expectorant. Topically – neuralgia, skin disorders; premature ejaculation. Topically, essential oil in aromatherapy – for nicotine withdrawal, skin conditions.

Safety in pregnancy: Appears safe in amounts commonly used in foods. AVOID ORAL THERAPEUTIC DOSES IN PREGNANCY – uterotonic. Caution: insufficient information on the safety of oral use when breastfeeding. Essential oil, topically and by inhalation – controversy over safety, but most authorities advise avoiding during pregnancy and breastfeeding; may be abortifacient. Potential contracting effects on uterine muscle suggest caution in labour and with postnatal lochial discharges.

Contraindications and precautions: Caution: insufficient information on safety in therapeutic doses. Do not confuse with Dong quai.

Adverse effects: Orally – constipation. Essential oil, topically – photosensitivity.

Interactions: Therapeutic oral doses, prolonged, excessive or inappropriate use may interact with amitriptyline, clozapine, diazepam, oestradiol, ondansetron, propranolol, theophylline, verapamil, warfarin. Oestrogenic herbs: black cohosh, blue cohosh, dong quai, evening primrose, fennel, fenugreek, ginkgo, ginseng, liquorice, raspberry leaf, red clover, vitex agnus castus. Also melatonin.

ANISE *see* **Aniseed**

ANISEED
Pimpinella anisum Herbal remedy, also known as Anise.

Indications: Orally – to increase lactation, induce menstruation, facilitate birth, increase libido, for dysmenorrhoea. Also for indigestion and flatulence, as an expectorant, diuretic, appetite stimulant. Topically – for psoriasis, lice, scabies.

Safety in pregnancy: Appears safe orally in amounts commonly found in foods and in small amounts topically. AVOID ORAL THERAPEUTIC DOSES IN PREGNANCY except under the supervision of a qualified medical herbalist.

Contraindications and precautions: Diabetes mellitus. Avoid if sensitive to plants in the Apiaceae family: asparagus, caraway, celery, coriander, cumin, dill, fennel. Avoid with hormone-sensitive conditions: breast, cervical and ovarian cancer, endometriosis, fibroids. Do not confuse with Star anise. Caution with commercial products containing aniseed and liquorice root.

Adverse effects: May lower blood glucose; may have anti-oestrogenic effects.

Interactions: Therapeutic oral doses, prolonged, excessive or inappropriate use may interact with contraceptive Pill, hormone replacement therapy, tamoxifen, antidiabetic medication, caffeine, diazepam, fluoxetine, imipramine and other tricyclic antidepressants. Oestrogenic herbs: black cohosh, blue cohosh, dong quai, evening primrose, fennel, fenugreek, ginkgo, ginseng, liquorice, raspberry leaf, red clover, vitex agnus castus. Hypoglycaemic herbs: devil's claw, fenugreek, Panax ginseng, Siberian ginseng. Herbs that interact with antidepressants: echinacea, ginkgo, ginseng, St John's wort.

ARABIC GUM *see* Acacia

ARBOR VITAE *see* Thuja

ARNICA
Arnica montana Herbal remedy, also known as Leopard's bane.

Indications: Orally – as an abortifacient. Also for mouth, throat inflammation, postoperative pain, swelling, bleeding, tooth extraction, insect bites, bruising. Topically, oil used for bruises, aches, sprains, insect bites, osteoarthritis, acne.

Safety in pregnancy: AVOID ORAL OR TOPICAL USE IN PREGNANCY, LABOUR AND POSTNATALLY – toxic, may cause miscarriage, antepartum haemorrhage, preterm labour, excessive lochial discharges, especially with retained products of conception.

Contraindications and precautions: Do not confuse with homeopathic Arnica.

Adverse effects: Hypertension, gastrointestinal tract irritation; dyspnoea, palpitations, nausea. Allergic reactions; anaphylaxis in those allergic to the Compositae family – daisies, marigolds, ragweed, etc. Toxic in large amounts – may cause miscarriage, hypertension, visual disturbance, sight loss, multiple organ failure, coma, death. Reports of herbal doses used to initiate miscarriage (abortion) causing multiple organ failure.

Interactions: Therapeutic oral doses, prolonged, excessive or inappropriate use may interact with anticoagulants and antiplatelet drugs: heparin, warfarin, aspirin, diclofenac, ibuprofen, enoxaparin. Anticoagulant herbs: angelica, clove, garlic, ginger, ginkgo, meadowsweet, Panax ginseng, poplar, red clover, turmeric.

ARNICA
Arnica montana Homeopathic remedy, from Leopard's bane.

Obstetric indications: Bruising; emotional and physical shock. Soft tissue trauma, for example perineal trauma after delivery. Postnatal afterpains. Bleeding gums. Labour – spasmodic, irregular, weak, ineffective contractions, occur with fetal movement; sharp, unbearable pain, stretched, traumatized muscles and tissues. Prolonged labour, retained placenta, retention of urine. Post-Caesarean pain and trauma. Neonatal – shock, especially after prolonged labour, instrumental delivery and caput succedaneum/cephalhaematoma. Available as tablets in different potencies and as cream.

Key features: Sore, swollen, bruised tissue; aching pain; joint and muscle pain; body feels battered and beaten; restless due to discomfort in any position; cold extremities but hot head; symptoms of physical shock; whole body sensitive; blunt trauma; haematoma formation.

Emotional symptoms: Very distressed but prefers to be left alone: "I'm all right"; fear of being touched or approached; dreams of accident or injury; poor concentration and memory.

Better for: Lying with head lower than feet; lying down.

Worse for: Cold; damp; touch; rest; movement.

Safety: Advised postnatal dose after physiological birth – one 30c tablet three times daily for 3–4 days, then STOP to avoid reverse proving. To increase dose, for example for instrumental or operative delivery, increase *frequency* of dose rather than number of tablets at each administration. After Caesarean section, Staphysagria may be preferable (incisive rather than blunt trauma) – do not use both unless under the supervision of a qualified homeopath. Topical application may cause skin irritation, allergic eczema, itching or dry, scaly skin; do not apply cream to open wounds. Do not use if there are any medical or obstetric complications. Not to be used as a replacement for standard medical care. Do not use with aromatherapy essential oils, topically or by inhalation, or with antacids, decongestants, laxatives or cough lozenges – inactivates the remedy. Do not take with food or drink. Do not take prophylactically – may lead to reverse proving. Should not be used by women who do not fit the symptom picture to avoid reverse proving. To be handled by the intended recipient only. Do not confuse with Arnica, the herbal remedy.

ARSENICUM

Arsenicum album Homeopathic remedy from metallic arsenic.

Obstetric indications: Food poisoning with nausea; profuse, often projectile, vomiting; diarrhoea. Carpal tunnel syndrome; cystitis; haemorrhoids; insomnia; indigestion; retention of urine; sore, cracked nipples. Contraction pain – sensation of burning with internal and external dryness.

Key features: Extreme exhaustion; weakness and faintness after minimal exertion. Chilly, with stinging pain like hot needles. Dryness, itchy and offensive, excoriating discharges. Nausea at the sight or smell of food; retching/profuse vomiting after eating/drinking; a bitter taste in the mouth. Wants cold food and drinks. Often abuse of alcohol/tobacco. Craves acid foods, coffee.

Emotional symptoms: Intense, selfish, perfectionist, demanding, organized, needs to be in control; wants reassurance about health; prone to phobias and obsessions. Tendency to monopolize people. Anxious, fastidious; fear of the unknown, suffocation, death.

Better for: Heat; warm food or drink; having head elevated; daytime; evening; sips of water; being in company.

Worse for: Lying down; between 0100–0200 hours; worse for becoming chilled; physical exercise; cold drinks or food; after eating; alcohol.

Safety: Arsenic occurs naturally in some foods such as seafood, poultry, mushrooms and some grains as a trace element. Do not confuse the homeopathic remedy with the full pharmacological doses of inorganic arsenic used in some Chinese medicines. Cases of arsenic poisoning from poorly prepared homeopathic arsenicum have been reported in India. Purchase it from a homeopathic pharmacy or a qualified homeopathic practitioner. Do not use if there are any medical or obstetric complications. Not to be used as a replacement for standard medical care. Do not use with aromatherapy essential oils, topically or by inhalation, or with antacids, decongestants, laxatives or cough lozenges – inactivates the remedy. Do not take with food or drink. Do not take prophylactically – may lead to reverse proving with serious toxic effects. Should not be used by women who do not fit the symptom picture to avoid reverse proving. To be handled by the intended recipient only.

ASHWAGANDHA

Withania somnifera, Physalis somnifera Herbal remedy, also known as Indian ginseng or Poison gooseberry.

Indications: Orally – for menstrual disorders, infertility (female and male), female sexual dysfunction, as an aphrodisiac, emmenagogue. Also for anxiety disorders, cognitive function, bipolar disorder, stress, attention deficit-hyperactivity disorder, insomnia, obsessive-compulsive disorder, arthritis, diabetes mellitus, cancer, chemotherapy-related fatigue. Used in Ayurvedic medicine.

Safety in pregnancy: AVOID IN PRECONCEPTION PERIOD, DURING MEDICAL INFERTILITY TREATMENT AND PREGNANCY – emmenagoguic, abortifacient.

Contraindications and precautions: Hypertension, hypotension, diabetes mellitus, thyroid conditions. Do not confuse with winter cherry (*Physalis alkekengi*).

Adverse effects: Nausea, vomiting, diarrhoea, heartburn, flatulence, skin irritation, headache, drowsiness.

Interactions: Antihypertensives, antidiabetic medication, benzodiazepines, barbiturates, immunosuppressants, thyroid medication. Antihypertensive herbs: cat's claw, coenzyme Q10, fish oil, stinging nettle. Sedative herbs: calamus, California poppy, catnip, hops, Jamaican dogwood, kava, St John's wort, skullcap, valerian, yerba mansa.

ASIAN GINSENG *see* **Ginseng**

ASTHMA PLANT *see* **Euphorbia**

ASTRALGUS
Astragalus membranaceus Herbal remedy, also known as Huáng qi.

Indications: Orally – for menopausal symptoms. Also for common cold, hay fever, fibromyalgia, anaemia, angina, asthma, immune system disorders, chronic fatigue, renal conditions, diabetes, infections. Topically – for wound healing. May be used intravenously by some qualified medical herbalists for cancers, leukaemia, immunocompromised conditions. Frequently used in traditional Chinese medicine.

Safety in pregnancy: AVOID REMEDIES DERIVED FROM ROOT, ORALLY OR TOPICALLY, IN PREGNANCY AND CHILDBIRTH – animal studies suggest maternal and fetal toxicity, although there is no evidence in humans.

Contraindications and precautions: Autoimmune conditions, peptic ulcer, diabetes mellitus, haemophilia, renal, hepatic disease. Do not confuse with Ma huang.

Adverse effects: Skin irritation. High doses may cause immunosuppression.

Interactions: Therapeutic oral doses, prolonged, excessive or inappropriate use may interact with immunosuppressants and lithium. Herbs with possible effects on immune system: berberine, cannabis, ginger, liquorice, turmeric.

BABOON URINE
Also known as Umchamo wemfene.

Indications: Traditional remedy in southern Africa as an aphrodisiac, to aid conception, reduce antenatal oedema, prepare for birth, aid labour progress. Appears to be available as commercially produced capsules.

Safety in pregnancy: Thought to increase uterine contractions, increasing the risk of miscarriage, preterm labour, precipitate labour, hypertonic uterine action in term labour. Advise extreme caution: AVOID UNTIL LATE THIRD TRIMESTER, caution in labour.

Contraindications and precautions: Avoid with previous Caesarean section, history of precipitate labour, preterm labour, well-established physiological labour.

Adverse effects: Sociological risk – several reports of men objecting to women's covert use as an aphrodisiac, resulting in domestic violence. Possible risk of infection from use of pure baboon urine rather than commercially prepared products.

Interactions: None documented, but advice is to avoid with uterotonic and oestrogenic drugs.

BARBERRY

Berberis vulgaris Herbal remedy, also known as European barberry.

Indications: Orally – for respiratory conditions, heartburn, colic, constipation, poor appetite, backache, hyperlipidaemia, diabetes mellitus, opioid withdrawal, renal, hepatobiliary conditions, as a vitamin C supplement. Topically – for bacterial vaginosis. Gel used in toothpaste for dental plaque and gingivitis.

Safety in pregnancy: AVOID THERAPEUTIC ORAL DOSES IN PREGNANCY AND BREASTFEEDING – contains berberine, thought to cross the placenta; may cause kernicterus in neonates.

Contraindications and precautions: Avoid with hypotension, haemorrhagic and coagulation disorders, diabetes mellitus. Do not confuse with Bearberry (Uva ursi). See also Berberine.

Adverse effects: Nausea, vomiting, headache, hypotension, hypertension, bradycardia, respiratory failure.

Interactions: Therapeutic oral doses, prolonged, excessive or inappropriate use may interact with anticoagulant and antiplatelet drugs, antidiabetic medication, benzodiazepines, tricyclic antidepressants, morphine. Anticoagulant herbs: angelica, clove, garlic, ginger, ginkgo, Panax ginseng, turmeric, willow bark. Hypoglycaemic herbs: bitter melon, fenugreek, ginger, goat's rue, kudzu. Hypotensive herbs: cat's claw, coenzyme Q10, stinging nettle. Sedative herbs: calamus, California poppy, catnip, hops, Jamaican dogwood, kava, melatonin, sage, St John's wort, sassafras, skullcap.

BASIL

Ocimum basilicum Herbal remedy, also known as Sabja, Tukmaria.

Indications: Orally – to stimulate circulation before and after labour; to stimulate lactation. Also for headaches, constipation, diarrhoea, common cold, kidney conditions, parasitic infections. In Ayurvedic and Chinese medicine, seeds are chewed as a nutritional supplement – they contain vitamins, minerals, fibre, flavonoids. Topically – essential oil in aromatherapy used to aid mental alertness, for anxiety, digestion, muscular pain. By inhalation, essential oil is used for upper respiratory tract infections.

Safety in pregnancy: Appears safe in amounts commonly used in foods. DO NOT USE THERAPEUTIC ORAL DOSES OR TOPICAL USE OF ESSENTIAL OIL IN PREGNANCY AND LACTATION – estragole content may be mutagenic.

Contraindications and precautions: Do not confuse with Holy basil.

Adverse effects: Excessive or prolonged oral use may cause liver damage. Topically – contact dermatitis. Estragole and its metabolites may be carcinogenic.

Interactions: Therapeutic oral doses, prolonged, excessive or inappropriate use may interact with anticoagulants: heparin, warfarin, aspirin, diclofenac, ibuprofen, enoxaparin. May also interact with antihypertensives. Anticoagulant herbs: angelica, clove, garlic, ginger, ginkgo, meadowsweet, Panax ginseng, poplar, red clover, turmeric. Hypotensive herbs: cat's claw, coenzyme Q10, fish oil, stinging nettle.

BEARBERRY *see* **Uva ursi**

BEE POLLEN
Animal product.

Indications: Orally – for premenstrual syndrome, menopausal and breast cancer-related hot flushes. Also as an appetite stimulant, to improve stamina, for hay fever, allergic rhinitis, dysuria, weight loss, haematemesis, epistaxis, constipation, diarrhoea, alcohol intoxication. Topically – for eczema, nappy rash.

Safety in pregnancy: AVOID ORALLY IN PREGNANCY AND EARLY POSTNATAL PERIOD – may have uterine-contracting effects.

Contraindications and precautions: Avoid with pollen allergies. Do not confuse with bee venom, honey, Royal jelly.

Adverse effects: Allergic reactions – itching, swelling, shortness of breath, dizziness, anaphylaxis. Long-term use may cause gastrointestinal and neurological symptoms.

Interactions: Therapeutic oral doses, prolonged, excessive or inappropriate use may interact with anticoagulants and anticoagulant herbs: angelica, clove, garlic, ginger, ginkgo, meadowsweet, Panax ginseng, poplar, red clover, turmeric.

BELLADONNA
Atropa belladonna Herbal remedy, also known as Deadly nightshade.

Indications: Orally – as a sedative, for bronchial asthma, common cold, hay fever, intestinal colic, inflammatory bowel disease, motion sickness. Topically – for rheumatism, sciatica, neuralgia; mental health issues. Rectally – for haemorrhoids.

Safety in pregnancy: AVOID IN PREGNANCY, LABOUR, POSTNATALLY AND FOR NEONATES – highly toxic. Secreted in breast milk; may impair lactation.

Contraindications and precautions: Constipation, hyperpyrexia, hypertension, oesophageal reflux, gastrointestinal ulcers or infections, ulcerative colitis, hiatus hernia, urinary retention, psychosis, cardiac disease. Do not confuse with Belladonna, the homeopathic remedy.

Adverse effects: Large amounts orally – atropine content may cause anticholinergic effects – muscle tremor, dilated pupils, tachycardia, hypertension or hypotension, disorientation, memory loss, hallucinations, confusion, psychosis, seizures, coma, respiratory failure.

Interactions: Therapeutic oral doses, prolonged, excessive or inappropriate use may interact with anticholinergic drugs: antihistamines, phenothiazines, tricyclic antidepressants. Anticholinergic herbs: henbane, ma huang, mandrake.

BELLADONNA
Atropa belladonna Homeopathic remedy from Deadly nightshade.

Obstetric indications: Backache in pregnancy, with a dragging sensation; excessive Braxton Hicks contractions; insomnia. Acute fever; headache/migraine; sore throat. Slow labour with poor cervical effacement, spasmodic and ineffectual contractions. Pain severe; bursting; throbbing from the sacrum to the thighs and from one hip to the other. Postnatally, engorged breasts, hard, red and inflamed, with red streaks; throbbing pain; over-abundant milk supply. Infant teething – painful, hot, red swollen cheeks, making the baby restless.

Key features: High temperature, flushed face and skin, pounding headaches or migraine; wide, glaring eyes, dilated pupils and localized inflammation, red and hot. Pulsating sensation; violent throbbing or spasms of muscular tissue. Throbbing carotid artery; right-sided symptoms.

Emotional symptoms: Irritable, restless, excitable, violent outbursts of rage; moaning with pain; fear of dogs and water; feels weak, exhausted and wants to escape.

Better for: Warmth; rest; sitting or standing upright; lying in a darkened room; pressure applied to head, cold compresses.

Worse for: Noise; touch; light, movement; lying down; cold draught; 1500 hours; swallowing food or drinks.

Safety: Since 2010, the US FDA has discouraged the use of homeopathic teething products containing belladonna. Although they may contain only homeopathic (trace) amounts of belladonna, there have been over 400 adverse reports of belladonna toxicity in babies, including seizures, dyspnoea, lethargy, constipation, difficulty urinating, agitation, and even death. For general safety do not use if there are any medical or obstetric complications. Not to be used as a replacement for standard medical care. Do not use with aromatherapy essential oils, topically or by inhalation, or with antacids, decongestants, laxatives or cough lozenges – inactivates the remedy. Do not take with food or drink. Do not take prophylactically – may lead to reverse proving. Should not be used by women who do not fit the symptom picture to avoid reverse proving. To be handled by the intended recipient only. Do not confuse with Belladonna, the herbal remedy.

BELLIS PERENNIS

Homeopathic remedy from Wild daisy.

Obstetric indications: Sudden abdominal and groin pain in pregnancy; sore uterus and stiffness in the lower abdomen. Muscle strain and sprains; deep muscular bruising after childbirth.

Key features: Weakness; bruised sensation often due to blows to soft tissue, post-surgery or strain to weak muscles; venous stasis; tired; left-sided symptoms; sleeplessness at 0300 hours; head pain from occiput to sinciput; stomach weak; nausea; loss of appetite. Pain – bruised, sore, squeezed sensation, sometimes triggered by sudden cold soaking.

Emotional symptoms: Tired, wishes to lie down, but prone to insomnia (wakes too early, cannot sleep again); angry dreams.

Better for: Rest and warmth; continuous motion; supporting the affected part.

Worse for: Becoming chilled when hot; touch; exertion; cold drinks when overheated; left side.

Safety: Do not use if there are any medical or obstetric complications. Not to be used as a replacement for standard medical care. Do not use with aromatherapy essential oils, topically or by inhalation, or with antacids, decongestants, laxatives or cough lozenges – inactivates the remedy. Do not take with food or drink. Do not take prophylactically – may lead to reverse proving. Should not be used by women who do not fit the symptom picture to avoid reverse proving. To be handled by the intended recipient only. Do not confuse with Wild daisy (*Bellis perennis*), herbal remedy.

BERBERINE

Berberine Herbal remedy from alkaloid in roots of plants including Barberry, Goldenseal, greater celandine, tree turmeric.

Indications: Orally – for polycystic ovary syndrome, menopausal symptoms. Also for irritable bowel syndrome, diarrhoea, *Helicobacter pylori* infection, diabetes mellitus, hypertension, hepatitis B and C, obesity, osteoporosis, cardiac conditions, stroke. Topically – for burns and sores. As eye drops – for glaucoma, chlamydial eye infection.

Safety in pregnancy: AVOID ORAL USE IN PREGNANCY AND BREASTFEEDING – crosses the placenta; may be teratogenic. Thought to stimulate smooth muscle – risk of miscarriage, preterm labour, hypertonic uterine contractions in term labour, excessive lochial discharges, especially with retained placenta. Neonates exposed to maternal berberine use via breast milk have been found to develop kernicterus.

Contraindications and precautions: Avoid in diabetes mellitus – may lower blood glucose levels; hypotension. Contraindicated in neonates; avoid during breastfeeding. Do not confuse with Barberry (*Berberis vulgaris*).

Adverse effects: Orally – diarrhoea, constipation, flatulence, vomiting, abdominal pain and distension, skin rash, headache. May affect liver function.

Interactions: Therapeutic oral doses, prolonged, excessive or inappropriate use may interact with anticoagulants and antiplatelet drugs: heparin, warfarin, aspirin, enoxaparin. May also interact with antidiabetic medication and antihypertensives: cyclosporine, diclofenac, tamoxifen, phenytoin, ondansetron. Herbs: angelica, bitter melon, California poppy, catnip, cat's claw, coenzyme Q10, chromium, clove, devil's claw, fenugreek, garlic, ginger, ginkgo, hops, horse chestnut, kava, Jamaican dogwood, melatonin, Panax ginseng, psyllium, sage, St John's wort, sassafras, Siberian ginseng, skullcap, stinging nettle. Also probiotics.

BERGAMOT

Citrus bergamia, *Citrus aurantium* Herbal remedy.

Indications: Essential oil, topically or by inhalation in aromatherapy – for relaxation, anxiety, stress, uplifting and mood enhancing, constipation, nausea, vomiting, flatulence, loss of appetite, pain relief, mild to moderate hypertension, insomnia. Orally – to reduce the side effects of antipsychotics and aromatase inhibitors for schizophrenia.

Safety in pregnancy: Essential oil used in aromatherapy appears safe in doses up to 1.5% in pregnancy and 2% in labour and the postnatal period.

Contraindications and precautions: Essential oil, topically or by inhalation in aromatherapy – avoid in women who are allergic to citrus fruit. Avoid exposure of skin to direct sunlight for at least 2 hours after topical use; discontinue if skin is itching. Do not ingest. Do not use neat on skin or directly in a birthing pool. Do not apply directly to breasts in postnatal period or wash with water before the baby starts feeding to avoid adverse neonatal effects from ingestion. Use a diffuser for a maximum of 15–20 minutes in any hour; do not vaporize in the second stage of labour to avoid neonatal exposure. Do not diffuse near neonates, the elderly, ill people or those who are allergic to citrus fruit. Do not diffuse in public areas or use excessive amounts that spread to public areas of a maternity unit, to avoid excessive exposure of the woman, baby, visitors and staff to potential adverse effects. Discontinue if any allergic reactions occur to avoid accumulative reaction to specific chemicals – may lead to anaphylactic shock in severe cases. Avoid prolonged use – furanocoumarins may cause malignant skin changes. Do not use with or store near homeopathic remedies. Store in a refrigerator to avoid rapid oxidation – shelf life of 3–6 months.

Adverse effects: Skin irritation if applied neat; photosensitivity. Orally – heartburn; potentially carcinogenic with prolonged use.

Interactions: Therapeutic oral doses, theoretically, prolonged, excessive or inappropriate use of essential oil may interact with anticoagulants or drugs with a similar action and also drugs with a photosensitizing effect. Anticoagulant herbs: angelica, clove, garlic, ginger, ginkgo, meadowsweet, Panax ginseng, poplar, red clover, turmeric.

BITTER ALMOND
Prunus amygdalus, Amygdalus communis Herbal remedy.

Indications: Orally – as an antispasmodic, local anaesthetic, narcotic, cough suppressant, antipruritic. Topically – for striae gravidarum, used as carrier oil in massage and aromatherapy.

Safety in pregnancy: AVOID ORAL USE IN PREGNANCY – contains toxic benzyl aldehyde and amygdalin, the latter metabolizing to potentially fatal hydrocyanic acid, thought to cause birth defects. Topically – appears safe enough, but advise caution.

Contraindications and precautions: Do not use topically for perineal massage or baby massage. Avoid oral use prior to general anaesthesia due to potential central nervous system depression. Do not confuse with Sweet almond.

Adverse effects: None reported with cautious use. Ingestion of oil from almond kernels may cause fatal respiratory and central nervous system depression due to hydrocyanic acid content (prussic acid), a by-product of which is cyanide.

Interactions: Therapeutic oral doses, prolonged, excessive or inappropriate use may interact with central nervous system depressants. Herbs affecting central nervous system: ginkgo, kava, ma huang, St John's wort, valerian.

BITTER KOLA *see* Gotu kola

BITTER ORANGE *see* ORANGE, Bitter

BLACK COHOSH
Cimicifuga racemosa, Actaea racemosa Herbal remedy.

Indications: Orally – for menopausal symptoms, induction of labour, infertility, premenstrual syndrome, dysmenorrhoea, infertility, breast cancer. Also for heartburn, anxiety, fever, sore throat, cough, cardiovascular disease, cognitive function, osteoarthritis, osteoporosis. Topically – for acne, skin conditioner, insect repellent, snake bites.

Safety in pregnancy: AVOID IN PREGNANCY BEFORE TERM. Appears safe enough for post-dates pregnancy or in labour to aid contractions. Caution in postnatal period if retained products of conception – uterotonic effects may precipitate secondary postpartum haemorrhage. Caution when breastfeeding – may have adverse hormonal effect on neonates.

Contraindications and precautions: Avoid with liver compromise, obstetric cholestasis. Avoid concomitant use with hormone replacement therapy or a history of oestrogen-dependent conditions – ovarian, breast and cervical cancer, endometriosis, fibroids. Do not use in physiologically normal term labour once contractions are established. Do not use with oxytocic drugs or other herbs thought to stimulate uterine contractions – Raspberry leaf, Evening primrose oil, Blue cohosh. Do not confuse with Blue cohosh. Question women about self-administration of herbal remedies to initiate labour and record in notes. Do not confuse with homeopathic Cimicifuga.

Adverse effects: Orally – breast tenderness, vaginal bleeding, gastrointestinal disturbance, skin rashes and irritation, headache, dizziness, cramping, hypotension, tiredness, irritability. Long-term use may be hepatotoxic, although evidence is minimal.

Interactions: Therapeutic oral doses, prolonged, excessive or inappropriate use may interact with carbamazepine, methyldopa and other hepatotoxic drugs, also amitriptyline, codeine, imipramine and ondansetron. Hepatotoxic herbs: comfrey, kava, pennyroyal oil, red yeast. May interfere with liver function test results. Oestrogenic herbs: angelica, blue cohosh, dong quai, evening primrose, fennel, fenugreek, ginkgo, ginseng, liquorice, raspberry leaf, red clover, vitex agnus castus.

BLACK HAW
Viburnum prunifolium Herbal remedy.

Indications: Orally – as a uterine relaxant to prevent miscarriage; for postnatal uterine involution, dysmenorrhoea. Also as a diuretic, antispasmodic, for diarrhoea, asthma. Often used interchangeably with Cramp bark.

Safety in pregnancy: AVOID IN PREGNANCY AND LABOUR – may be a uterine relaxant; teratogenic. Safe in therapeutic doses to treat miscarriage under the supervision of a qualified medical herbalist.

Contraindications and precautions: Avoid with a history of renal calculi – oxalic acid content may increase stone formation. Avoid with aspirin allergy or asthma.

Adverse effects: May reduce iron, zinc, calcium absorption.

Interactions: Therapeutic oral doses, prolonged, excessive or inappropriate use may interact with aspirin and herbs containing salicylate: aspen bark, meadowsweet, poplar, willow bark.

BLACK HENBANE *see* Henbane

BLACK MUSTARD

Brassica nigra Herbal remedy.

Indications: Orally – for common cold, rheumatism, osteoarthritis, to induce vomiting, as a diuretic, appetite stimulant. Topically – oil used as a poultice for respiratory disorders, joint and muscle pain.

Safety in pregnancy: Appears safe in amounts commonly used in foods. AVOID THERAPEUTIC ORAL DOSES IN PREGNANCY – may be abortifacient, potentially causing miscarriage, preterm labour. Caution: no information available on safety during breastfeeding.

Contraindications and precautions: Avoid in those sensitive to mustard or other members of the Brassicaceae family – cabbage, broccoli, turnips, kale. Do not use oil for baby massage; seeds are not suitable for children under six. Do not confuse with white mustard.

Adverse effects: Orally – allergic reactions including oral mucosal irritation. High dietary consumption may cause or exacerbate cardiac, gastric and hepatic effects. Inhalation of ground mustard may cause respiratory irritation. Topically – increased sensitivity to pain, burns, toxic dermatitis. May interfere with blood glucose.

Interactions: Therapeutic oral doses, prolonged, excessive or inappropriate use may interact with diabetic medication and hypoglycaemic herbs: devil's claw, fenugreek, Panax ginseng, Siberian ginseng.

BLACK PEPPER

Piper nigrum Herbal remedy, essential oil.

Indications: Orally – for dysmenorrhoea, pain relief in labour. Also for constipation, diarrhoea, oedema, depression, fatigue, headache, reduced libido; asthma, bronchitis, rhinitis, sinusitis; weight loss. Topically as an essential oil in aromatherapy – for backache, pain relief in labour, a stimulant. By inhalation – for smoking cessation, swallowing dysfunction.

Safety in pregnancy: Appears safe in amounts commonly used in foods. Some suggest that large oral doses may be abortifacient. Topically, essential oil appears safe in pregnancy in doses up to 1.5% and in labour and postnatally in doses up to 2%.

Contraindications and precautions: Topically – avoid if there is pyrexia: rubefacient. Do not diffuse – overpowering aroma may cause respiratory reactions. Do not ingest. Do not use neat on skin or directly in a birthing pool. Discontinue use if any allergic reactions occur to avoid accumulative reaction to specific chemicals – may lead to anaphylactic shock in severe cases. Store in a refrigerator; do not use with or store near homeopathic remedies. Orally in therapeutic doses – caution in diabetes as may affect serum glucose. Avoid with haemorrhagic disorders, prior to surgery – may cause bleeding, bruising.

Adverse effects: Orally – heartburn, allergic reactions. Topically – skin irritation, photosensitivity. By inhalation – cough, redness of eyes.

Interactions: Therapeutic oral doses, prolonged, excessive or inappropriate use may interact with anticoagulant and antiplatelet drugs: heparin, warfarin, aspirin, diclofenac, ibuprofen, enoxaparin. May also interact with antidiabetic medication and certain antidepressants: amoxycillin, codeine, ondansetron, loperamide, carbamazepine, cyclosporine, theophylline, verapamil, propranolol. Herbs: angelica, clove, devil's claw, dong quai, fenugreek, garlic, ginger, ginkgo, meadowsweet, Panax ginseng, poplar, red clover, Scotch broom, Siberian ginseng, turmeric.

BLACK SEED *see* Nigella

BLOND PSYLLIUM *see* Ispaghula

BLOODROOT
Sanguinaria canadensis Herbal remedy.

Indications: Orally – for bronchitis, asthma, laryngitis, constipation, irritable bowel syndrome, nasal polyps, warts, to induce vomiting. Topically – as a dental analgesic.

Safety in pregnancy: AVOID ORAL OR TOPICAL USE IN PREGNANCY AND BREASTFEEDING – contains sanguinarine, a toxic alkaloid.

Contraindications and precautions: Avoid with gastrointestinal inflammatory conditions, glaucoma. Do not confuse with Bloodwort/Yarrow.

Adverse effects: Orally – nausea, vomiting, central nervous system depression, glaucoma, hypotension, shock, coma. Topically – contact dermatitis.

Interactions: None documented, but in view of potential adverse effects advice is to avoid therapeutic oral doses and prolonged, excessive or inappropriate use with antihypertensives and central nervous system depressants.

BLUE CHAMOMILE *see* Chamomile, German

BLUE COHOSH
Caulophyllum thalictroides Herbal remedy.

Indications: Orally – popular remedy for induction of labour, to stimulate menstruation, for uterine inflammation, pelvic inflammatory disease, endometriosis. Also for constipation, colic, sore throat, cramps, hysteria.

Safety in pregnancy: AVOID IN PREGNANCY AND LABOUR – teratogenic, mutagenic. Caulosaponin glycoside content may cause vasoconstriction and oxytocic activity leading to miscarriage in early pregnancy, preterm labour or hypertonic uterine action at term. Controversy over safety to induce/accelerate labour – many US midwives traditionally use blue cohosh, but increasing safety concerns have reduced its use. UK and Canadian herbalists strongly advise against use in pregnancy and labour unless under the supervision of an experienced medical herbalist. N-methylcytosine content may have nicotine-like effects. Anagyrine content may impact on maternal cardiac muscle, potentially causing hypertension and cardiac arrhythmias. Question women about self-administration of herbal remedies to initiate labour and record in notes. Advise women to avoid ALL products containing herbal blue cohosh in preconception, antenatal, intrapartum and early postnatal periods.

Contraindications and precautions: Avoid in hormone-sensitive conditions due to possible oestrogenic effects – breast, uterine and ovarian cancer, endometriosis, uterine fibroids. Do not use in well-established term labour or with oxytocic drugs to expedite labour. Avoid with hypertension, diabetes mellitus, irritable bowel syndrome. Do not confuse with herbal Black cohosh, homeopathic Caulophyllum or homeopathic Cimicifuga.

Adverse effects: Therapeutic doses immediately before or during labour may cause hypertonic uterine action, leading to fetal distress and meconium-stained liquor. Excessive maternal use may cause headache, nausea, diarrhoea, mucous membrane irritation, tachycardia, sweating, abdominal pain, vomiting, hyponatraemia, hyperglycaemia, hypertension, muscle twitching, hypotension, hepatotoxicity, cardiotoxicity. Maternal consumption near term may cause fetal hypertension, hyperglycaemia or neonatal respiratory distress, renal failure, convulsions, acute myocardial infarction, congestive heart failure, cerebrovascular accident.

Interactions: Therapeutic oral doses, prolonged, excessive or inappropriate use may interact with antidiabetic medication or antihypertensives: frusemide, nicotine. Hypoglycaemic herbs: devil's claw, fenugreek, Panax ginseng, Siberian ginseng. Hypotensive herbs: basil, cardamom, celery seed, cinnamon, flaxseed, garlic, ginger, hawthorn. Oestrogenic herbs: black cohosh, dong quai, evening primrose, fennel, fenugreek, ginkgo, ginseng, liquorice, raspberry leaf, red clover, vitex agnus castus.

BLUE GUM *see* Eucalyptus

BLUE PIMPERNEL *see* Skullcap

BLUE VERVAIN *see* Verbena

BORAGE
Borago officinalis Herbal remedy.

Indications: Orally – for premenstrual syndrome, menopausal symptoms, to initiate labour, promote lactation, for neonatal prematurity. Also for stress, depression, diabetes mellitus, attention deficit-hyperactivity disorder, alcoholism, asthma, as a diuretic or sedative. Topically – for eczema, seborrheic dermatitis. Mainly used as oil from crushed seeds, commercially prepared as capsules.

Safety in pregnancy: Appears safe in amounts commonly used in foods. AVOID THERAPEUTIC DOSES IN PREGNANCY AND BREASTFEEDING – some borage-containing products contain hepatotoxic-pyrrolizidine alkaloids when taken orally; may also be carcinogenic, mutagenic or teratogenic with long-term use. Pyrrolizidine alkaloids excreted in breast milk – may increase risk of kernicterus in jaundiced babies.

Contraindications and precautions: Advise women to avoid commercial borage preparations unless labelled as free of hepatotoxic-pyrrolizidine alkaloids. Do not use commercially prepared capsules intravaginally to initiate labour at term; avoid excessive consumption of tea at term. Discontinue use at least two weeks before elective surgery. Avoid with coagulation disorders, liver compromise including obstetric cholestasis, schizophrenia.

Adverse effects: Orally – diarrhoea, flatulence. Excessive or prolonged ingestion of products containing pyrrolizidine alkaloids – hepatotoxicity, carcinogenicity, mutagenicity, toxic to respiratory system; may increase platelet and cholesterol levels.

Interactions: Therapeutic oral doses, prolonged, excessive or inappropriate use may interact with anticoagulant and antiplatelet drugs: heparin, warfarin, aspirin, enoxaparin. May also interact with non-steroidal anti-inflammatories: diclofenac, ibuprofen, naproxen, phenothiazines. Anticoagulant herbs: angelica, clove, garlic, ginger, ginkgo, meadowsweet, Panax ginseng, poplar, red clover, turmeric. Hepatotoxic herbs: agrimony, butterbur, coltsfoot, comfrey, golden ragwort, hemp, tansy ragwort. Also echinacea, garlic, liquorice, St John's wort, schisandra. May prolong bleeding time and affect tests for clotting factors in susceptible women.

BRAZIL ROOT *see* Ipecacuanha, herbal remedy

BROMELAIN
Ananas comosus, Ananas ananas Herbal remedy, Pineapple.

Indications: Orally – popular remedy from enzymes in the core of fresh, raw pineapple, to stimulate labour onset. Also therapeutic doses used orally for postoperative swelling and pain, allergic rhinitis, smooth muscle relaxation and/or contraction, renal calculi, to facilitate antibiotic absorption, increase fat excretion, for ulcerative colitis, rheumatoid arthritis.

Safety in pregnancy: Appears safe to eat in moderate amounts, although pineapple is considered a "forbidden fruit" in many countries. Known to impact on smooth muscle, but stimulatory or relaxation effects appear dose-dependent. Occurs in the central fibrous stem and core of fresh raw pineapple, and is destroyed by cooking, canning or juicing. To ingest sufficient bromelain from pineapple to trigger uterine contractions, several complete pineapples would need to be consumed: a therapeutic dose of commercially prepared bromelain is likely to be more effective, although evidence for its impact on smooth muscle is inconclusive.

Contraindications and precautions: AVOID IN THERAPEUTIC DOSES UNTIL TERM. Advise women to avoid excessive consumption of pineapple or commercially prepared bromelain tablets if any pregnancy, maternal or fetal complications. Question women about self-administration of herbal remedies to initiate labour and record in notes. Avoid if due for elective Caesarean section – risk of bleeding. Avoid if there is a latex or pineapple allergy possible or in those who experience lip tingling when eating raw pineapple.

Adverse effects: Allergic skin reactions – urticaria, pruritis, swelling. Excessive consumption may cause diarrhoea, nausea, vomiting, abdominal pain. Serious allergic reactions, including anaphylaxis, in those who are allergic to pineapple. Long-term consumption can cause protein breakdown, possibly leading to haemorrhage.

Interactions: Therapeutic oral doses, prolonged, excessive or inappropriate use may interact with anticoagulants and antiplatelet drugs: heparin, warfarin, aspirin, diclofenac, ibuprofen, enoxaparin. May also interact with amoxycillin. Anticoagulant herbs: alfalfa, angelica, aniseed, arnica, asafoetida, celery, chamomile, clove, fenugreek, feverfew, garlic, ginger, horse chestnut, liquorice, meadowsweet, poplar, red clover, willow. Theoretically, concomitant consumption of potato or soybeans may reduce the therapeutic effects of bromelain due to chemicals that inhibit proteolytic enzymes.

BRYONIA

Bryonia alba Homeopathic remedy from white bryony.

Obstetric indications: Abdominal/back pain with stiffness. Breast pain in pregnancy; postnatally engorged breasts, which are hard, hot but pale and painful, an over-abundant milk supply. Constipation, with large, dry, hard stools; flatulence, heartburn; watery, bitter-tasting vomit. Vulval varicosities. Key remedy for a dry cough, influenza.

Key features: Slow onset of symptoms. Pain – stitch-like, stabbing on the slightest movement; may grasp painful part for support. Bursting, splitting headache; vertigo when head is raised. Excessive thirst; dry mucous membranes – lips, mouth and eyes; bitter taste; feeling of a stone in the stomach. Irritating dry, hacking cough with dyspnoea.

Emotional symptoms: Angry, anxious or apathetic. Needs to be left alone, very irritable when disturbed. Worry about finances and being away from home whilst unwell. Feels mentally dull; cannot explain what they want. Hopelessness, worrying dreams; fear of death.

Better for: Cool air; firm pressure and lying on affected parts; lying down; staying still; cold drinks.

Worse for: Slightest movement; bright lights; noise; light touch; after eating; warm environment; stooping; between 2100–0300 hours.

Safety: Incompatible with homeopathic Calcarea carbonica. Do not use if there are any medical or obstetric complications. Not to be used as a replacement for standard medical care. Do not use with aromatherapy essential oils, topically or by inhalation, or with antacids, decongestants, laxatives or cough lozenges – inactivates the remedy. Do not take with food or drink. Do not take prophylactically – may lead to reverse proving. Should not be used by women who do not fit the symptom picture to avoid reverse proving. To be handled by the intended recipient only. Do not confuse with White bryony/Bryonia, the herbal remedy.

CABBAGE

Brassica oleracea Herbal remedy.

Indications: Topically – to relieve oedema; popular remedy to reduce postnatal breast engorgement. Orally – for gastrointestinal disorders, pregnancy sickness, to prevent osteoporosis and certain cancers.

Safety in pregnancy: Topically – appears safe for short-term use. Excessive postnatal consumption of cabbage can cause colic in breastfed babies.

Contraindications and precautions: Avoid oral and topical use in those sensitive to the Brassicaceae plant family – broccoli, Brussels sprouts, cauliflower, horseradish, mustard, radish, turnip, etc. Contains significant amounts of vitamin K – risk of coagulation disorders with excessive oral consumption. Should not be consumed orally in excessive amounts in those with diabetes mellitus – may decrease serum glucose. Avoid oral therapeutic doses with thyroid disorders – antithyroid constituents may increase thyroid-stimulating hormone levels.

Adverse effects: Topically – skin irritation, contact dermatitis (rare). Orally in excessive amounts – diarrhoea, bruising, bleeding, hypoglycaemia. May interfere with tests for clotting factors, serum glucose, thyroid hormones.

Interactions: Therapeutic oral doses, prolonged, excessive or inappropriate oral use may interact with antidiabetic medication, paracetamol, anticoagulants, especially warfarin, and antiplatelet drugs: pentazocine, morphine, clozapine, imipramine. Hypoglycaemic herbs: devil's claw, fenugreek, garlic, horse chestnut, Panax ginseng, psyllium, Siberian ginseng. Anticoagulant herbs: alfalfa, angelica, aniseed, chamomile, clove, fenugreek, feverfew, garlic, ginger, horse chestnut, liquorice, meadowsweet, poplar, red clover, turmeric, willow bark.

CACTUS *see* **Hoodia**

CALABASH CHALK
Mineral product, also known as Calabar stone, Mabele or Nzu.

Indications: Orally – traditionally consumed for pregnancy sickness, hypersalivation. Also as a nutritional supplement and for recreational use, primarily amongst Nigerian and other West African communities.

Safety in pregnancy: AVOID IN PRECONCEPTION PERIOD, PREGNANCY AND BREASTFEEDING – may contain high lead and arsenic levels that impair general reproductive function (in men also), and cause intrauterine growth retardation, low birth weight and poor mental development of neonates. In the UK, Public Health England has advised against its use since 2013. Animal studies suggest possible impairment of maternal antenatal weight gain. Breastfeeding: apparently safe enough if already consuming when breastfeeding commenced, but advise women not to (re)commence consumption whilst breastfeeding.

Contraindications and precautions: Do not confuse with American calabash tree. Clay product, called Sikor or Shikor mati, used for similar purposes, should also not be consumed in pregnancy.

Adverse effects: Toxicity – high lead, arsenic, aluminium levels may affect infant neurological development. Alterations in haemoglobin, red blood cell levels, erythrocyte sedimentation rate; poor absorption of iron and zinc from nutrients; intestinal blockage; demineralization of femur bone.

Interactions: None documented, but given identified adverse effects, advice is to avoid concomitant use with iron, vitamin and mineral therapy.

CALCAREA CARBONICA
Homeopathic remedy, tissue salt from carbonate of lime.

Obstetric indications: Low backache, especially from lifting. Carpal tunnel syndrome with tingling, numbness, oedema of wrists/fingers. Constipation with clay-like stools, followed by diarrhoea. Flatulence, indigestion and heartburn with bloated abdomen and pressing pain. Insomnia before midnight, overactive mind and anxious dreams. Nausea worse with milk, sour vomiting like curdled milk. Prolonged, intermittent postnatal lochia, with milky appearance. Poor milk supply, full breasts, sometimes sore. Pain – cutting, pulsating, stitching, griping.

Key features: Catches cold easily, malaise; lethargy, easily fatigued, sluggish. Profuse foot perspiration (offensive) and head; right-sided symptoms. Swollen lymphatics, bloated, heavy sensation, burning vaginal irritation, with candida infection. Craves salt, sweet, indigestible foods, raw potato. Generally prone to kidney and gallstones, uterine fibroids.

Emotional symptoms: Dislikes getting wet; hates being observed. Poor concentration, difficulty in verbal expression and confusion; lacks initiative; irrational fears of insanity and other people's views; over-concentration on trivialities; sad, irritable, obstinate.

Better for: Dry climate; warmth; lying down; lying on painful side; after breakfast.

Worse for: Exertion; cold, raw air; ascending movement; milk; waking; night-time; wet weather; bathing; after eating; thinking about condition.

Safety: Generally used for constitutional conditions (those to which the individual's constitution is predisposed) rather than acute conditions; rarely causes a healing reaction. Should not be given before homeopathic sulphur; incompatible with homeopathic Bryonia. Do not use if there are any medical or obstetric complications. Not to be used as a replacement for standard medical care. Do not use with aromatherapy essential oils, topically or by inhalation, or with antacids, decongestants, laxatives or cough lozenges – inactivates the remedy. Do not take with food or drink. Do not take prophylactically – may lead to reverse proving. Should not be used by women who do not fit the symptom picture to avoid reverse proving. To be handled by the intended recipient only.

CALENDULA

Calendula officinalis Herbal remedy, also sometimes known as Marigold.

Indications: Orally – to initiate menstruation, for dysmenorrhoea, as an antispasmodic. Also to reduce fever, oral and pharyngeal inflammation, for gastric and duodenal ulcer, headache, jaundice. Topically – for inflammation, wound healing, burns, nosebleeds, varicose veins, haemorrhoids, gingivitis, nappy rash, sore nipples, vaginal candidiasis. Essential oil used as an insect repellent. Available as commercially produced cream.

Safety in pregnancy: Topical use appears safe. AVOID THERAPEUTIC DOSES ORALLY IN PRECONCEPTION PERIOD AND PREGNANCY – abortifacient, spermicidal, may interfere with implantation of blastocyst.

Contraindications and precautions: Avoid oral and dermal use in those who are sensitive to plants in the Asteraceae/Compositae family – ragweed, chrysanthemums, marigolds, daisies. If cream is used for sore nipples, advise washing nipples with plain water prior to feeding the baby. Do not confuse with homeopathic Calendula. Do not confuse with Marigold of the *Tagetes* genus.

Adverse effects: Orally – allergic reactions, theoretical risk of anaphylaxis but very few recorded cases. Topically – eczematous skin reactions, especially if sensitive to chrysanthemums, marigolds, daisies, etc.

Interactions: Therapeutic oral doses, prolonged, excessive or inappropriate use may interact with sedatives and central nervous system depressants. Sedative and central nervous system depressant herbs: calamus, California poppy, ginkgo, hops,

Jamaican dogwood, kava, ma huang, melatonin, sage, St John's wort, sassafras, skullcap, valerian.

CALENDULA

Calendula officinale Homeopathic remedy from calendula.

Obstetric indications: Wounds, cuts, lacerations, perineal trauma, sore nipples. Infection of umbilical cord. Useful after tooth extraction.

Key features: Grazed, torn, ragged wounds; abscesses; suppurating wounds; inflammation; redness; chilly. Pain – out of proportion to presenting problem, feels as if beaten; exhausted. Renowned for antiseptic properties, acts on epithelial tissue to promote granulation.

Emotional symptoms: Extremely nervous and frightened.

Better for: Warmth; rest.

Worse for: Cloudy, heavy, damp weather; evening.

Safety: Do not use if there are any medical or obstetric complications. Not to be used as a replacement for standard medical care. Do not use with aromatherapy essential oils, topically or by inhalation, or with antacids, decongestants, laxatives or cough lozenges – inactivates the remedy. Do not take with food or drink. Do not take prophylactically – may lead to reverse proving. Should not be used by women who do not fit the symptom picture to avoid reverse proving. To be handled by the intended recipient only. Do not confuse with herbal Calendula or herbal Marigold.

CANNABIS

Cannabis sativa Herbal remedy, also known as Hemp, Marijuana or Dagga.

Indications: By inhalation – for nausea and vomiting, including pregnancy sickness, appetite stimulation, insomnia, various chronic conditions and life-limiting illnesses. Orally – for pain relief, particularly in chronic or life-limiting conditions, for example multiple sclerosis. Also smoked for recreational purposes.

Safety in pregnancy: AVOID IN PRECONCEPTION PERIOD, PREGNANCY AND BREASTFEEDING. Contains over 100 cannabinoids that pass to the fetus via the placenta and to neonates in breast milk. Associated with miscarriage, gestational hypertension, intrauterine growth retardation, preterm labour, placental abruption, stillbirth, low birth weight, maternal or childhood anaemia, maternal psychosis, learning difficulties and psychotic episodes in the child. During breastfeeding, cannabis is stored in adipose tissue; THC[1] can remain in

---

1   Tetrahydrocannabinol (THC) is one of at least 113 cannabinoids identified in cannabis and is the principal psychoactive constituent of cannabis.

breast milk for up to six days, potentially causing delayed cerebral development in the baby.

Contraindications and precautions: Caution with women presenting with hyperemesis gravidarum – regular or excessive use may lead to cannabinoid hyperemesis syndrome. Avoid if allergic to peaches, tomatoes, Mugwort, bananas, citrus fruit. Avoid confusion with hemp that contains much less psychoactive THC than pure cannabis and is generally considered safer, although caution urged in pregnancy and breastfeeding.

Adverse effects: Smoking – headache, dizziness, drowsiness, fatigue, dry mouth, nausea, increased appetite, allergic reactions, immunosuppression. Hyper- or hypotension, tachycardia, palpitations, major cardiovascular conditions. Paranoia, psychosis, dyspnoea, hallucinations, panic attacks, depression, reduced motor coordination and reaction times, poor memory. Epileptiform fits and cannabinoid hyperemesis syndrome – intractable vomiting unrelieved by conventional medication, possibly leading to serious complications such as Wernicke's encephalopathy, renal, cardiac, hepatic failure, degeneration of skeletal muscle, death. Increased risk of lung cancer with prolonged smoking.

Interactions: Oral administration, recreational smoking and inhalation; prolonged, excessive or inappropriate use may interact with anaesthetics, anticoagulants and antiplatelet drugs: heparin, warfarin, aspirin, diclofenac, ibuprofen, enoxaparin. Anticoagulant herbs: angelica, clove, garlic, ginger, ginkgo, meadowsweet, Panax ginseng, poplar, red clover, turmeric. Sedative herbs: calamus, California poppy, catnip, hops, Jamaican dogwood, kava, St John's wort, skullcap, valerian, yerba mansa. Also alcohol.

CARBO VEGETALIS

Homeopathic remedy, tissue salt from wood charcoal, sometimes called "death remedy".

Obstetric indications: Complete exhaustion in labour, fainting; collapse due to oxygen starvation. Failure to progress in labour; contractions very weak, tearing, pressing, constricting, moving from the groin to the legs, then ceasing completely. Neonatal resuscitation. Also for indigestion; heartburn and flatulence.

Key features: Weakness; faintness; fatigue; physical and mental exhaustion; extreme weariness on minimal activity; icy cold body; sluggish. Cold, clammy externally, but feels hot internally. Indigestion, trapped offensive wind, abdominal bloating. Air hunger with oxygen starvation. Specific feature – may say they have fully recovered from previous illness or accident. Craves alcohol, junk food, coffee, sweets, salty food.

Emotional symptoms: Mentally sluggish, poor concentration, poor memory; indifferent, sad, tearful; anxiety at night; fears the supernatural.

Better for: Cool, fresh air; being fanned; belching.

Worse for: Fatty food; coffee, milk, wine; in the evening; warm, damp weather; lying down.

Safety: Should not be administered for neonatal resuscitation at birth unless under the close supervision of a qualified homeopath in attendance with a midwife or doctor. Do not use if there are any medical or obstetric complications. Not to be used as a replacement for standard medical care. Do not use with aromatherapy essential oils, topically or by inhalation, or with antacids, decongestants, laxatives or cough lozenges – inactivates the remedy. Do not take with food or drink. Do not take prophylactically – may lead to reverse proving. Should not be used by women who do not fit the symptom picture to avoid reverse proving. To be handled by the intended recipient only.

CASCARA
Frangula purshiana Herbal remedy, also known as African coffee tree.

Indications: Orally – primarily for constipation, also gallstones and hepatic conditions.

Safety in pregnancy: AVOID IN PREGNANCY AND BREASTFEEDING – too purgative; indirect effect of excessive peristalsis may cause uterine contractions leading to miscarriage, preterm labour. Excreted in breast milk, may cause diarrhoea in a neonate.

Contraindications and precautions: Avoid with gastrointestinal conditions, for example ulcerative colitis; do not use long term. Do not confuse with Cascarilla (Cinchona).

Adverse effects: Maternal/neonatal diarrhoea, abdominal cramps, vomiting. Long-term use – potassium depletion, electrolyte disturbance, proteinuria, haematuria, muscle weakness, impaired cardiac function.

Interactions: Therapeutic oral doses, prolonged, excessive or inappropriate use may interact with laxatives, diuretics and steroids. Laxative herbs: alder buckthorn, aloe, black root, blue flag, butternut bark, European buckthorn, greater bindweed, rhubarb, senna, yellow dock. Also bilberry, black hellebore, brewer's yeast, Canadian hemp root, digitalis leaf, figwort, hedge mustard, horsetail, lily of the valley root, liquorice, motherwort, oleander leaf, pleurisy root.

CASCARILLA *see* Cinchona

CASSAVA *see* Yucca

CASTOR OIL
Ricinus communis Herbal remedy from the castor bean.

Indications: Orally – common remedy to stimulate labour; also for constipation, to promote lactation, as a contraceptive. Topically – for skin disorders, abscess, headache, ear inflammation. Intracervically as an abortifacient. In some African countries, the seeds are crushed and extracted oil is drunk during labour to prevent perineal lacerations (called Mupfuta).

Safety in pregnancy: AVOID IN PREGNANCY BEFORE TERM – very purgative, may cause excessive diarrhoea, indirectly contributing to miscarriage, preterm labour. If used to stimulate term/post-dates labour, should be under the supervision of a midwife, doctor or qualified medical herbalist. Question women about their use of herbal remedies to initiate labour and record in notes.

Contraindications and precautions: Do not use in conjunction with other pharmacological methods to induce labour – Black cohosh, Blue cohosh, Evening primrose oil, Raspberry leaf, oxytocic drugs, administered orally, vaginally or intravenously. Do not exceed single dose of 60ml. Do not consume uncoated whole seeds. Avoid hulled seeds with hypertension. Avoid oil with gastrointestinal conditions, for example ulcerative colitis, hypersensitivity conditions, symptoms of appendicitis, rectal fissures.

Adverse effects: Orally – miscarriage, preterm labour; excessive use at term may cause incoordinate, painful or hypertonic uterine action, fetal distress and meconium-stained liquor. Abdominal discomfort, cramping, diarrhoea, nausea, faintness. Chewing uncoated castor bean seeds can be fatal due to ricin content (a substance used in germ warfare). Topically – skin irritation. Excessive or prolonged consumption – potassium loss leading to hypokalaemia.

Interactions: Therapeutic oral doses, prolonged, excessive or inappropriate use may interact with oxytocic drugs, cervical ripening agents, diuretics and laxatives. Herbal laxatives: chamomile, dandelion, ginger, liquorice, marshmallow, peppermint, senna. Advise caution with oestrogenic herbs: black cohosh, blue cohosh, dong quai, evening primrose, fennel, fenugreek, ginkgo, ginseng, liquorice, raspberry leaf, red clover, vitex agnus castus.

CAULOPHYLLUM

Caulophyllum thalictroides Homeopathic remedy from Blue cohosh.

Obstetric indications: Late onset of labour. Failure to progress in labour – short, distressing, irregular, ineffectual contractions causing the woman to cry out in agony. Atonic uterus, rigid cervical os with poor effacement and dilatation; stalled labour from exhaustion. Contractions intermittent, cramping, spasmodic, felt in the groin and legs, flitting from one place to another; accompanied by needle-like pain in the cervix. Irritability, with exhaustion, trembling, feeling chilly.

Key features: Generalized and muscular weakness; fever but feels cold; thirsty; faintness and internal trembling; nausea with the sensation of fullness in the epigastric area; profuse, vaginal discharge; rheumatic aches in small joints.

Emotional symptoms: Nervous exhaustion; anxious, fretful, apprehensive and irritable; can barely move or speak due to extreme weakness (out of proportion to pain and weakness). In post-dates pregnancy may appear to be "hanging on" to pregnancy, not "letting go".

Better for: Pressure; lying on the left side.

Worse for: Hot weather; lying on the back or right side.

Safety: May be inappropriately used to stimulate labour onset – most effective for women who do not want to "let go" and allow the body to start labour or for those with poor muscle tone and a history of difficult labour. Routine or prophylactic caulophyllum taken as birth preparation in the last weeks of pregnancy may seriously disturb uterine polarity due to reverse proving, causing either very short, violent precipitate labour or, conversely, protracted labour. Do not use with pharmacological oxytocics to expedite labour, including medically prescribed drugs and herbal remedies such as Raspberry leaf, Evening primrose oil, Clary sage, Black cohosh and Blue cohosh. Compares closely with homeopathic Cimicifuga – physiology similar but emotionally different – cautious use to avoid reverse proving from inappropriate use. Do not use if there are any medical or obstetric complications. Not to be used as a replacement for standard medical care. Do not use with aromatherapy essential oils, topically or by inhalation, or with antacids, decongestants, laxatives or cough lozenges – inactivates the remedy. Do not take with food or drink. Do not take prophylactically – may lead to reverse proving. Should not be used by women who do not fit the symptom picture to avoid reverse proving. To be handled by the intended recipient only. Do not confuse with herbal Blue cohosh (*Caulophyllum thalictroides*).

CAUSTICUM

Causticum Hahnemannii Homeopathic remedy, tissue salt from potassium hydrate.

Obstetric indications: Constipation with ineffectual desire to defecate; cystitis or postpartum retention of urine, with frequent, painful, ineffectual desire to urinate. Also for heartburn, ligament pain, cramp. Pain – tearing, burning, stitch-like, itching.

Key features: Lack of coordination, restless legs at night, progressive weakness/paralysis of muscles, trembling, debility, indescribable fatigue, heaviness of body and eyelids; loss of voice or stammering; cracks and skin eruptions, thick, copious catarrh. Desires smoked meat, salt, beer; dislikes sweet foods.

Emotional symptoms: Worries, mental weariness, over-concern for friends/family/business matters; introverted and timid, suspicious, pessimistic, quarrelsome; fears darkness and dogs.

Better for: Warm, wet weather; cold drinks; gentle motion; warmth.

Worse for: Cold, dry weather; long-standing grief or anxiety; loss of sleep; night; mental or physical exertion; fright; twilight; thinking about complaints; fatty food; right side.

Safety: Do not use in conjunction with homeopathic phosphorous or Coffea. Do not use if any medical or obstetric complications. Not to be used as a replacement for standard medical care. Do not use with aromatherapy essential oils, topically or by inhalation, or with antacids, decongestants, laxatives or cough lozenges – inactivates the remedy. Do not take with food or drink. Do not take prophylactically – may lead to reverse proving. Should not be used by women who do not fit the symptom picture to avoid reverse proving. To be handled by the intended recipient only.

CEDAR LEAF *see* Thuja

CHAMOMILE, German
Matricaria chamomilla Herbal remedy, also known as Blue chamomile.

Indications: Orally – for dysmenorrhoea. Also for flatulence, hay fever, diarrhoea, anxiety, restlessness, insomnia, gastrointestinal colic, heartburn, inflammatory bowel disease, peptic ulcer. Topically – for wound healing, haemorrhoids, mastalgia, vaginal inflammation, leg ulcers, eczema, gingivitis. Essential oil by inhalation – respiratory conditions.

Safety in pregnancy: AVOID ORAL USE OF THERAPEUTIC DOSES AND TOPICAL USE OF ESSENTIAL OIL IN PREGNANCY AND LABOUR. May cause miscarriage due to phytoestrogen content; AVOID IN BREASTFEEDING except as commercially prepared topical ointment for sore nipples.

Contraindications and precautions: Orally – avoid in those sensitive to the Asteraceae/Compositae family – ragweed, chrysanthemums, marigolds, daisies. Caution with chamomile tea, may contain either German or Roman chamomile. Avoid excessive doses when used for insomnia – may cause mental over-stimulation, wakefulness. Avoid if history of hormone-sensitive conditions – breast, uterine and ovarian cancer, endometriosis, uterine fibroids. Avoid prior to general anaesthetic – possible effects on the central nervous system. Essential oil, topically and by inhalation – avoid until postnatal period; Roman chamomile is preferable. Avoid with respiratory conditions. Store in a refrigerator to avoid rapid oxidation. Do not confuse with Roman chamomile. Do not confuse with homeopathic Chamomilla.

Adverse effects: Orally – allergic reactions including severe hypersensitivity reactions, possibly leading to anaphylaxis. Topically – allergic contact dermatitis, eczema. By inhalation – respiratory reactions, eye irritation. May reduce urinary creatinine.

Interactions: Therapeutic oral doses, prolonged, excessive or inappropriate use may interact with anticoagulants and antiplatelet drugs: heparin, warfarin, aspirin.

May also interact with non-steroidal anti-inflammatories: ibuprofen and naproxen. Also sedatives, benzodiazepines, ondansetron, fentanyl, theophylline, oestrogens, tamoxifen, contraceptive Pill, tricyclic antidepressants, chlorpromazine, alcohol. Anticoagulant herbs: angelica, clove, garlic, ginger, ginkgo, meadowsweet, Panax ginseng, poplar, red clover. Sedative herbs: calamus, California poppy, catnip, hops, kava, St John's wort, saw palmetto, skullcap, valerian, yerba mansa. Oestrogenic herbs: black cohosh, blue cohosh, dong quai, evening primrose, fennel, fenugreek, ginkgo, ginseng, liquorice, raspberry leaf, red clover, vitex agnus castus.

CHAMOMILE, Roman
Chamaemelum nobile, Anthemis nobilis Herbal remedy.

Indications: Topically – as essential oil in aromatherapy for dysmenorrhoea, premenstrual syndrome pregnancy sickness, constipation, indigestion, heartburn, flatulence, irritable bowel syndrome, loss of appetite, inflammation, wound healing, cracked nipples, skin conditions, haemorrhoids. By inhalation – for sinusitis, hay fever, ear inflammation. Orally as tea – for insomnia, relaxation.

Safety in pregnancy: Essential oil appears safe for topical use in aromatherapy in doses up to 1.5% in pregnancy and 2% in labour, postnatally. Avoid oral therapeutic doses in pregnancy; may cause threatened miscarriage, preterm labour, risk of lower infant birth weight. Tea generally considered safe in moderate amounts.

Contraindications and precautions: Orally and by inhalation – avoid if sensitive to plants in the Asteraceae/Compositae family – ragweed, chrysanthemums, marigolds, daisies – or with known skin sensitivities. Avoid oral therapeutic doses in haemorrhagic disorders or prior to surgery – may cause bleeding, bruising. Caution with chamomile tea, may contain either German or Roman chamomile – avoid excessive doses when used for insomnia – may cause mental over-stimulation, inability to sleep. Essential oil in aromatherapy – do not ingest. Do not use neat on skin or directly in a birthing pool. Do not apply directly to breasts in postnatal period, or wash with water before the baby starts feeding to avoid adverse neonatal effects from ingestion. Use a diffuser for a maximum of 15–20 minutes in any hour; do not vaporize in the second stage of labour to avoid neonatal exposure; do not diffuse near neonates, elderly or ill people. Do not diffuse in public areas or use excessive amounts which spread to public areas of maternity unit, to avoid excessive exposure of the woman, baby, visitors and staff to potential adverse effects. Discontinue use if any allergic reactions occur to avoid accumulative reaction to specific chemicals – may lead to anaphylactic shock in severe cases. Store in a refrigerator to avoid rapid oxidation. Do not use with or store near homeopathic remedies. Do not confuse with German chamomile, herbal remedy, or Chamomilla, homeopathic remedy.

Adverse effects: Excessive oral consumption may cause vomiting. Excessive consumption of tea may cause irritation, agitation, prevent sleep. Topically –

contact dermatitis, eczema. Respiratory allergic reactions, from both inhalation and topical use.

Interactions: Therapeutic oral doses, prolonged, excessive or inappropriate use may interact with sedatives and sedative herbs: calamus, California poppy, catnip, hops, kava, St John's wort, saw palmetto, skullcap, valerian, yerba mansa.

CHAMOMILLA

Matricaria chamomilla Homeopathic remedy from German chamomile.

Obstetric indications: Labour – failure to progress. Contractions severe, unbearable, distressing but very weak, eventually cease; pain – cutting, tearing, pulsating, pressing upwards. Postnatal afterpains – unbearable, with bad temper. Insomnia due to pain, anger, stimulants or excessive consumption of Chamomile tea, even in infants; vivid dreams. Infant teething with unbearable pain, cries out in sleep; cheeks hot and red or pale and cold with red spot on one cheek; often with diarrhoea, green stools.

Key features: Low pain threshold, intolerant of pain, notably verbalizes "I can't bear it" or "I want to die". Hot, perspiring, thirsty but aversion to warm drinks; restless, red-faced; exhaustion; nausea; feels faint. Feels hot; if in bed, kicks off bedclothes and sticks "burning" feet out of bed. Loose stools, flatulence; acrid, offensive discharges; may rock backwards and forwards.

Emotional symptoms: Very bad tempered, hostile, impossible to please, quarrelsome, insensitive to others, angry and impatient due to pain, oversensitive to noise. Self-centred; wants attention but rejects it when offered. Baby whines, screams but cannot be comforted; older infants ask for things that they immediately throw (drinks, toys, etc.); they insist on being carried and cry when put down, taking parents to the limits of endurance.

Better for: Fresh air; passive movement; warm, wet weather.

Worse for: Anger; heat; cold, windy weather; noise; pain; from 2100 hours onwards; touch; consolation.

Safety: Ensure teething granules are purchased from a reputable company. Although chamomilla teething granules have not been found to contain toxic levels, some teething products may contain other homeopathic remedies, including Belladona, discouraged by the FDA in the USA. Do not use if there are any medical or obstetric complications. Not to be used as a replacement for standard medical care. Do not use with aromatherapy essential oils, topically or by inhalation, or with antacids, decongestants, laxatives or cough lozenges – inactivates the remedy. Do not take with food or drink. Do not take prophylactically – may lead to reverse proving. Should not be used by women who do not fit the symptom picture to avoid reverse proving. To be handled by the intended recipient only. Do not confuse with German chamomile or Roman chamomile, herbal remedies.

CHASTE BERRY, CHASTE TREE *see* **Vitex agnus castus**

CHIMARRAO *see* **Yerba mate**

CHINA *see* **Cinchona bark**

CHINA ROSE *see* **Hibiscus**

CHINESE ANGELICA *see* **Dong quai**

CHINESE GINSENG *see* **Ginseng**

CHINESE MOTHERWORT *see* **Motherwort**

CHINESE RHUBARB *see* **Rhubarb**

CHRYSANTHEMUM *see* **Tansy**

CIMICIFUGA

Cimicifuga racemosa Homeopathic remedy from black cohosh.

Obstetric indications: Key remedy for unbearable afterpains, worse in groin. Labour – late onset, with fear of birth. Ineffectual contractions – sharp, spasmodic, tearing, like electric shocks, irregular, fly in all directions around abdomen, back, hips; increase if cold, decrease if warm. Retained placenta, with shaking, trembling, exhaustion.

Key features: Cramping sensation in hips; trembling, chilly. May feel faint, blood pressure may be raised; heavy sensation in limbs; jerking; rheumatic aches and pains; muscular soreness following exertion, may lead to insomnia; sensations of numbness; top of head liable to fly off.

Emotional symptoms: Intense fears and emotional instability; fear of death, pain, the birth, going mad. Hysterical, talkative, fear of something bad about to happen; terrifying memories; restless; visions of mice and rats; "I can't do this"; feel like dark cloud overshadowing; very pessimistic and complaining.

Better for: Open air; bending double; gentle movement; warm wraps.

Worse for: Cold draughts; sitting, stress, noise and pain.

Safety: Compares closely with Caulophyllum – physiology similar, emotionally different – cautious use to avoid reverse proving from inappropriate use. Do not use if there are any medical or obstetric complications. Not to be used as a replacement for standard medical care. Do not use with aromatherapy essential oils, topically or by inhalation, or with antacids, decongestants, laxatives or cough lozenges – inactivates the remedy. Do not take with food or drink. Do not take prophylactically – may lead to reverse proving. Should not be used by women who do not fit the symptom picture to avoid reverse proving. To be handled by the intended recipient only. Do not confuse with Black cohosh or Blue cohosh, herbal remedies, or with Caulophyllum, homeopathic remedy.

CINCHONA

Cinchona officinalis Herbal remedy, also known as Cascarilla.

Indications: Orally – to stimulate appetite, promote salivary secretion, for haemorrhoids, varicose veins, leg cramps, influenza, mouth and throat conditions, muscle cramps, digestive disorders. Topically – for eye lotions, haemorrhoids, skin conditions, varicose veins, to stimulate hair growth.

Safety in pregnancy: AVOID ORAL AND TOPICAL USE IN PREGNANCY AND BREASTFEEDING – abortifacient, fetotoxic, teratogenic, passes to breast milk.

Contraindications and precautions: Avoid with gastrointestinal conditions, muscle wasting conditions. Do not confuse with homeopathic Cinchona bark. Do not confuse with Cascarilla (*Croton eluteria*) or Cascara.

Adverse effects: Orally – excessive or prolonged use may cause toxicity – nausea, vomiting, diarrhoea, tinnitus, visual disturbance, cardiac arrhythmias, haematological disorders, death. Topically – contact dermatitis.

Interactions: Therapeutic oral doses, prolonged, excessive or inappropriate use may interact with antacids, quinine, anticoagulant and antiplatelet drugs, carbamazepine, codeine, amitriptyline, fluoxetine, methadone, cimetidine, ranitidine. Anticoagulant herbs: alfalfa, angelica, clove, garlic, ginger, horse chestnut, Panax ginseng, red clover.

CINCHONA BARK

Cinchona officinalis Homeopathic remedy from cinchona bark, also known as China.

Obstetric indications: Diarrhoea in pregnancy, painless, stools with undigested food. Indigestion, bloated abdomen, bitter belching tasting of food eaten, pressing pain. Nervous exhaustion, with profuse sweating.

Key features: Poor appetite; dislikes bread and butter, fruit, rich fatty food; prefers cold drinks, spicy foods, sweets. Skin sore all over body, dislikes being touched. Profuse cold sweats on covered parts of body, increased with slightest exertion. Looks anaemic, weak, pale face with dark rings round eyes.

Emotional symptoms: Anxious, depressed, apathetic; does not like being touched. Fearful of dogs; sensitive to noise.

Better for: Firm pressure.

Worse for: Cold, fresh air; light touch; movement; at night.

Safety: Do not use if there are any medical or obstetric complications. Not to be used as a replacement for standard medical care. Do not use with aromatherapy essential oils, topically or by inhalation, or with antacids, decongestants, laxatives or cough lozenges – inactivates the remedy. Do not take with food or drink. Do not take prophylactically – may lead to reverse proving. Should not be used by women who do not fit the symptom picture to avoid reverse proving. To be handled by the intended recipient only. Do not confuse with Cinchona, herbal remedy.

CINNAMON

Cinnamomum verrum, Cinnamomum Zeylanicum Herbal remedy from Ceylon cinnamon.

Indications: Orally – for polycystic ovary syndrome, dysmenorrhoea. Also for irritable bowel syndrome, indigestion, diarrhoea, flatulence, diabetes mellitus and pre-diabetes, obesity, hay fever, common cold, cough, influenza; as a mouth rinse. Essential oil (produced from both cinnamon leaf and bark) – used topically or by inhalation in some countries to stimulate contractions at term. Commonly used in Ayurvedic medicine.

Safety in pregnancy: Appears safe in amounts commonly used in foods. AVOID THERAPEUTIC ORAL DOSES IN PREGNANCY – may be abortifacient. AVOID ESSENTIAL OIL USE IN PREGNANCY – uterine-stimulating effect may cause miscarriage, preterm labour. Appears safe, orally, topically and by inhalation, in doses up to 2% when breastfeeding.

Contraindications and precautions: Orally – avoid therapeutic doses in postnatal period with hypotension, pre-existing or gestational diabetes mellitus – risk of hypoglycaemia. Essential oil, topically and by inhalation – extremely powerful, use with caution in labour in doses up to maximum 1.5% *only* after 40 weeks' gestation, under the supervision of a qualified aromatherapist with experience of using in labour. Midwives and other birth workers not fully qualified in aromatherapy should not use it. AVOID IN WELL-ESTABLISHED PHYSIOLOGICAL LABOUR OR WITH OXYTOCICS – risk of uterine hyperstimulation. Not to be used by pregnant midwives or other birth attendants. Do not ingest. Do not use neat on skin or directly in a birthing pool. Do not apply directly to breasts in postnatal period, or wash with water before the baby starts feeding to avoid adverse neonatal effects from ingestion. Do not vaporize in labour to avoid neonatal exposure; do not diffuse in the postnatal period near neonates, elderly or ill people. Do not diffuse near animals – harmful to cats and dogs. Do not diffuse in public areas or use excessive amounts which spread to public areas of maternity unit, to avoid excessive exposure of the woman, baby, visitors and staff to potential adverse effects. Discontinue use if any allergic reactions occur to avoid accumulative reaction to specific chemicals – may lead to anaphylactic shock in severe cases. Store in a refrigerator to avoid rapid oxidation.

Do not use with or store near homeopathic remedies. Do not confuse with Cassia cinnamon that contains high levels of coumarins, increasing hepatotoxicity risk.

Adverse effects: Topically – significant risk of severe contact dermatitis, irritation of mucous membranes. Some essential oil suppliers recommend a skin patch test prior to use, although this may not be a realistic option in labour. Some companies will sell only to qualified aromatherapy practitioners. Excessive or prolonged respiratory or dermal administration may cause headache, dizziness, eye irritation, abdominal pain, diarrhoea. Orally – heartburn, nausea, bloating, indigestion, blood thinning, loss of consciousness.

Interactions: Therapeutic oral doses, prolonged, excessive or inappropriate dermal and respiratory essential oil use may interact with antidiabetic medication and antihypertensives. Hypoglycaemic herbs: bitter melon, chromium, devil's claw, fenugreek, garlic, guar gum, horse chestnut, Panax ginseng, psyllium, Siberian ginseng. Hypotensive herbs: cat's claw, coenzyme Q10, fish oil, stinging nettle.

CLARY SAGE
Salvia sclarea Herbal remedy.

Indications: Topically and by inhalation – essential oil popularly used to initiate labour, for retained placenta. Also for intrapartum pain relief, as a sedative, for depression, to improve mental function, reduce blood pressure. Herbal remedy orally – for digestive disturbance, renal disease.

Safety in pregnancy: AVOID THERAPEUTIC ORAL DOSES AND ESSENTIAL OIL, TOPICALLY OR BY INHALATION, UNTIL TERM, minimum 37 weeks' gestation. Advise women not to self-administer at home to initiate contractions – risk of hypertonic uterine action with injudicious use. Essential oil appears safe enough for use in maternity intrapartum aromatherapy *with caution*, in a maximum dose of 2%. Valuable when labour is not yet well established but consider effects comparable with oxytocin. Increasingly used inappropriately by many women desperate to start labour and by some midwives and doulas, leading to hypertonic uterine action, fetal distress. Over-use by maternity professionals can lead to disturbed uterine polarity, resulting in either hypertonic uterine action or, conversely, to reduced uterine action via negative feedback mechanism.

Contraindications and precautions: Do not use in well-established physiological labour – risk of hypertonic uterine action, fetal distress, meconium-stained liquor. Question women about self-administration of herbal remedies to initiate labour and record in notes. If used by midwives or doulas to accelerate stalled first stage labour, ensure no cephalopelvic disproportion and all other normal observations undertaken before use, for example check for hypoglycaemia, full bladder, pain, etc. – may be safer to use different essential oils to manage stress or pain to help re-establish effective uterine action. Avoid with uterine scar from previous Caesarean section, especially within the last two years. Avoid with intrapartum epidural anaesthesia; avoid in hypotensive women. Do not use concomitantly with oxytocin, dinoprostone or other drugs to stimulate contractions. Do not use for retained placenta if placenta is partially separated or lodged in the cervical canal – risk of severe primary postpartum haemorrhage. Avoid in postpartum period if retained products of conception – risk of secondary postpartum haemorrhage. Not to be used by pregnant midwives and other maternity staff or those who are trying to conceive or undergoing fertility treatment; avoid use for labouring woman if accompanied by a pregnant relative. May cause menorrhagia in menstruating staff. Do not ingest. Do not use neat on skin or directly in a birthing pool. Do not diffuse in labour or in public areas, or use excessive amounts which spread to public areas of maternity unit, to avoid excessive exposure of the woman, baby, visitors and staff to potential adverse effects. Discontinue use if any allergic reactions occur to avoid accumulative reaction to specific chemicals – may lead to anaphylactic shock in severe cases. Avoid if the mother is on antidepressants or antihypertensives. Store in a refrigerator – it oxides quickly. Do not use with or store near homeopathic remedies. Do not confuse with Sage (*Salvia officinale*).

Adverse effects: Emmenagoguic action – capable of causing menstruation-like vaginal bleeding in non-pregnant women, menorrhagia in menstruating women. Overdose or inappropriate use in pregnancy may cause miscarriage, preterm labour, hypertonic uterine contractions in labour or, conversely, reduction in uterine action – usually due to overdose from excessive or prolonged use, fetal distress, meconium-stained liquor, primary postpartum haemorrhage, excessive lochial discharge, secondary postpartum haemorrhage, usually from misuse. May reduce blood pressure, causing dizziness. Sedative action can cause headache with prolonged use – ensure judicious use in well-ventilated room to avoid becoming over-sedated, so staff can make clinical decisions in emergency situations. May potentiate the effects of alcohol – caution if maternity staff drink alcohol after prolonged occupational exposure to clary sage. High ketone content is thought to be neurotoxic and organotoxic. Skin irritation. May be adulterated with other substances containing linalool or linalyl acetate, either natural or synthetic – purchase good quality products with certification of purity. Note: There is very little direct evidence on clary sage; contraindications, precautions and adverse effects are extrapolated from considerable experiential evidence of significant use in maternity care.

Interactions: Therapeutic oral doses, prolonged, excessive or inappropriate dermal or inhalational use may interact with synthetic oxytocin- or prostaglandin-based drugs to stimulate uterine action; alcohol; antidepressants, antihypertensives, bupivacaine used in epidural anaesthesia. Oestrogenic herbs: black cohosh, blue cohosh, dong quai, evening primrose, fennel, fenugreek, ginkgo, ginseng, liquorice, raspberry leaf, red clover, vitex agnus castus.

CLOVE
Syzygium aromaticum Herbal remedy.

Indications: Orally – for indigestion, diarrhoea, halitosis, flatulence, nausea, vomiting, cough. Topically, essential oil, known as clove bud – for toothache, including infant teething, healing after tooth extraction, inflammation of mouth, throat, gums; for anal fissures; pruritus; premature ejaculation; as mosquito repellent. Herb occasionally smoked in conjunction with tobacco to numb airways and facilitate deeper nicotine inhalation.

Safety in pregnancy: Appears safe in amounts commonly used in foods. AVOID THERAPEUTIC DOSES ORALLY, AND ESSENTIAL OIL TOPICALLY OR BY INHALATION IN PREGNANCY – may be abortifacient, cause serious systemic effects. Caution: insufficient information available on safety when breastfeeding.

Contraindications and precautions: Essential oil, topically – do not use for infant teething: may cause mouth and gum irritation, sensitivity and damage tooth pulp of emerging teeth; swallowing oil can lead to fluid imbalance, convulsions, liver damage. Eugenol content may delay blood clotting – avoid with excessive postnatal lochia, haemorrhagic or clotting disorders. Do not smoke clove cigarettes – can cause respiratory difficulties; long-term use can lead to pulmonary disease. Do not diffuse essential oil or smoke near animals – harmful to cats and dogs.

Adverse effects: Orally in therapeutic doses – bleeding, bruising, hypoglycaemia, intravascular disseminated coagulation, metabolic acidosis, convulsions, hepatic failure, electrolyte imbalance, respiratory distress. As mouthwash – gum damage, irritation of mucous membranes, mouth ulcers. Topically – contact dermatitis, itching, rash, burning and tingling sensations. Inhalation of essential oil – itching, respiratory distress, pulmonary oedema, aspiration pneumonitis. Smoking – tachycardia, hypertension, increased serum nicotine, tar and carbon monoxide absorption.

Interactions: Therapeutic oral doses, prolonged, excessive or inappropriate use may interact with anticoagulants and antiplatelet drugs: heparin, warfarin, aspirin, diclofenac, ibuprofen, enoxaparin. Anticoagulant herbs: angelica, dong quai, garlic, ginger, ginkgo, horse chestnut, Panax ginseng, poplar, red clover, turmeric, willow bark.

CLUB MOSS

Lycopodium clavatum Herbal remedy, also known as Wolf's claw.

Indications: Orally – as diuretic, for urinary tract infections.

Safety in pregnancy: Very little information available on safety, but advise AVOID ORAL THERAPEUTIC DOSES IN PREGNANCY – contains toxic alkaloids, although no cases of poisoning documented.

Contraindications and precautions: Avoid with cardiovascular disease, lung disorders, gastrointestinal ulcers, epilepsy, urogenital conditions. Do not confuse with Lycopodium, homeopathic remedy. Do not confuse with *Lycopodium selago/ Huperzia selago* (Chinese club moss).

Adverse effects: Nausea, vomiting, abdominal discomfort, asthma. Serious cholinergic toxicity – nausea, dizziness, slurred speech, cramping – may be thought to be due to *Lycopodium clavatum* but is more likely to be due to *Huperzia selago* (Chinese club moss).

Interactions: Cholinergic, anticholinergic, acetylcholinesterase inhibitors. Cholinergic ashwagandha, holy basil, ginger, cinnamon. Anticholinergic herbs: belladonna, henbane.

COCCULUS

Cocculus indicus Homeopathic remedy from Indian berry, also known as levant berry.

Obstetric indications: Complete exhaustion, usually from irregular sleeping, as with night feeds. Headache, dizziness, insomnia. Pregnancy/travel sickness.

Key features: Aversion to fresh air. Hungry but dislikes food in general. Hot flushes. Trembling, with exhaustion, emotion. Sickness – specifically exacerbated by movement.

Emotional symptoms: Anxious, confused, dazed, forgetful, introspective. Grief or anger.

Better for: Lying down in bed.

Worse for: Exertion; loss of sleep; movement; touch; walking in fresh air.

Safety: Not suitable for hyperemesis gravidarum. Do not use if there are any medical or obstetric complications. Not to be used as a replacement for standard medical care. Do not use with aromatherapy essential oils, topically or by inhalation, or with antacids, decongestants, laxatives or cough lozenges – inactivates the remedy. Do not take with food or drink. Do not take prophylactically – may lead to reverse proving. Should not be used by women who do not fit the symptom picture to avoid reverse proving. To be handled by the intended recipient only. Do not confuse with Indian berry/levant berry, herbal remedy – toxic central nervous system and gastrointestinal irritant.

COENZYME Q10

Ubiquinol, Ubiquinone Naturally occurring fat-soluble compound, chemically similar to vitamin K.

Indications: Orally – for pre-eclampsia, male infertility, polycystic ovary syndrome. Also for coenzyme Q10 deficiency, cardiovascular and cardiac conditions, diabetes mellitus, hypertension, hyperlipidaemia, bipolar disorder, athletic performance, chronic fatigue syndrome, to stimulate immune system, for migraine, fibromyalgia, cocaine dependence, asthma, sepsis. Topically – for periodontal disease.

Safety in pregnancy: Appears safe in therapeutic doses in pregnancy and lactation.

Contraindications and precautions: Essential or gestational hypertension, abdominal disturbance.

Adverse effects: Nausea, vomiting, diarrhoea, appetite suppression, heartburn, epigastric discomfort (rare).

Interactions: Therapeutic oral doses, prolonged, excessive or inappropriate use may interact with antihypertensives and anticoagulants: heparin, warfarin, aspirin, diclofenac, ibuprofen, enoxaparin. Also beta-carotene, omega-3 fatty acids, vitamins A, C, E, K. Hypotensive herbs: cat's claw, coenzyme Q10, fish oil, stinging nettle. Also acacia, black pepper, red yeast rice.

COFFEA
Coffea cruda Homeopathic remedy from coffee.

Obstetric indications: Pain relief; insomnia; headaches.

Key features: Symptoms typical of over-stimulation, irritability from excess coffee consumption: restlessness, irritability, insomnia, acute senses; mind racing with thoughts, unable to switch off; one-sided headache, hypersensitive to pain. Contractions unbearable, irregular, worse in sacrum; ineffective. Pain – severe; tight; spasmodic.

Emotional symptoms: Euphoric or excited but despairing; talkative; cries out in pain; tearful and moaning; fears will go crazy, fears death.

Better for: Warmth; lying down; cold water; rest.

Worse for: Draughts; noise; odours; touch; tea or coffee; excessive emotions.

Safety: Do not use in conjunction with Causticum. Avoid drinking coffee while taking coffea. Do not use if there are any medical or obstetric complications. Not to be used as a replacement for standard medical care. Do not use with aromatherapy essential oils, topically or by inhalation, or with antacids, decongestants, laxatives or cough lozenges – inactivates the remedy. Do not take with food or drink. Do not take prophylactically – may lead to reverse proving. Should not be used by women who do not fit the symptom picture to avoid reverse proving. To be handled by the intended recipient only. Do not confuse with coffee.

COLA NUT
Cola acuminata, Sterculia acuminate Herbal remedy, also known as Kola nut.

Indications: Orally – for relief of mental and physical fatigue, depression, chronic fatigue syndrome, melancholy, weight loss, migraine headache.

Safety in pregnancy: Considered safe enough in pregnancy and breastfeeding but urge caution, avoid excessive consumption due to high caffeine levels. Has not been shown to be teratogenic.

Contraindications and precautions: Advise women to monitor overall caffeine intake including coffee, tea, cola, other caffeine-containing products. Excessive caffeine consumption associated with miscarriage, preterm labour, intrauterine growth retardation, low birth weight; may cause symptoms of caffeine withdrawal in neonates, including irritability and diarrhoea. Do not confuse with Gotu kola.

Adverse effects: Insomnia, anxiety, nervousness, gastrointestinal problems, tremors, mouth blisters and sensitivity. Extreme consumption may reduce bone density. Prolonged excessive consumption may cause crystalline retinopathy, anorexia. May affect tests for clotting factors, urinary catecholamines, vanillyl mandelic acid tests for phaeochromocytoma.

Interactions: Therapeutic oral doses, prolonged, excessive or inappropriate use may interact with alcohol, coffee, amphetamines, cocaine, ephedrine, nicotine, Ventolin, cimetidine, clozapine, contraceptive Pill, oestrogens, fluconazole, lithium, monoamine oxidase inhibitors, certain antibiotics, theophylline, antidiabetic medication. Also anticoagulants and antiplatelet drugs: heparin, warfarin, aspirin, diclofenac, ibuprofen, enoxaparin. Anticoagulant herbs: angelica, clove, garlic, ginger, ginkgo, Panax ginseng. Also ma huang, black tea, cocoa, coffee, green tea, oolong tea, guarana, yerba mate, bitter orange, calcium, magnesium, creatinine. Oestrogenic herbs: black cohosh, blue cohosh, dong quai, evening primrose, fennel, fenugreek, ginkgo, ginseng, liquorice, raspberry leaf, red clover, vitex agnus castus.

COLCHICUM

Colchicum autumnale Homeopathic remedy from autumn crocus.

Obstetric indications: Exhaustion, nausea and vomiting specifically with acute sense of smell. Also for diarrhoea, flatulence, joint pain.

Key features: Heightened sense of smell, including any cooked food, worse with egg. Sensitive to cold, damp, movement.

Emotional symptoms: Absent-minded, forgetful, sensitive to conflict.

Better for: Sitting down.

Worse for: Cold, damp weather, especially in autumn; night-time; sight of food.

Safety: Do not use if there are any medical or obstetric complications. Not to be used as a replacement for standard medical care. Do not use with aromatherapy essential oils, topically or by inhalation, or with antacids, decongestants, laxatives or cough lozenges – inactivates the remedy. Do not take with food or drink. Do not take prophylactically – may lead to reverse proving. Should not be used by women who do not fit the symptom picture to avoid reverse proving. To be handled by the intended recipient only. Do not confuse with autumn crocus, herbal remedy – mutagenic; colchicine content leads to acute poisoning.

COMFREY
Symphytum officinale Herbal remedy.

Indications: Orally – for menorrhagia, diarrhoea, haematuria, cough, bronchitis, gastritis, peptic ulcer, tuberculosis, cancer, angina. Topically – for wound healing, bruising, muscle soreness, back pain, leg ulcers, osteoarthritis, haemorrhoids, fractures.

Safety in pregnancy: AVOID ORAL AND TOPICAL USE IN PRECONCEPTION PERIOD, PREGNANCY, LABOUR, POSTNATAL PERIOD AND FOR NEONATES – teratogenic, hepatotoxic, carcinogenic.

Contraindications and precautions: Topically – avoid with liver compromise. Do not apply to broken skin – hepatotoxic-pyrrolizidine alkaloids absorbed through skin. Avoid oral use completely – risk of hepatotoxicity.

Adverse effects: Topically – skin redness, irritation, itching, eczema. Orally – hepatotoxic, may interfere with liver function tests; carcinogenic, mutagenic.

Interactions: Therapeutic oral doses, prolonged, excessive or inappropriate use may interact with carbamazepine, phenobarbital, phenytoin, methyldopa. Hepatotoxic herbs: agrimony, borage, echinacea, garlic, golden ragwort, hemp, kava, liquorice, St John's wort, schisandra.

COMMON MOTHERWORT *see* **Motherwort**

COWSLIP
Primula officinalis, Primula veris Herbal remedy.

Indications: Orally – for respiratory mucous membrane inflammation, cough, bronchitis, insomnia, headache, dizziness, hysteria, neuralgia, as diuretic, antispasmodic; for whooping cough, asthma, neurological complaints. Commercially available, often combined with gentian root, verbena, sorrel, elderflower or thyme.

Safety in pregnancy: Commercially available combination products appear safe enough in non-pregnant people. Little information available on safety in pregnancy and childbirth, avoid using, except under the supervision of a qualified medical herbalist.

Contraindications and precautions: Generally – avoid in those with gastrointestinal conditions.

Adverse effects: Gastrointestinal disturbance, allergic skin reactions.

Interactions: None specifically documented, although individual flavonoid constituents may interact with some drugs and herbs when taken in therapeutic doses.

CRAMP BARK
Viburnum opulus Herbal remedy.

Indications: Orally – for dysmenorrhoea, antenatal cramp, cramping contractions during labour, thought to prevent miscarriage and treat preterm labour through antispasmodic effect, inflammation of uterus. Also for cramps, muscle spasms, painful or spasmodic urinary conditions, nervous disorders, diuretic, emetic, purgative, sedative.

Safety in pregnancy: Appears safe in late pregnancy, but advise women to consult a qualified medical herbalist before use.

Contraindications and precautions: Avoid in aspirin sensitivity. Do not confuse with Black haw (*Vibernum prunifolium*), Cranberry, Uva ursi.

Adverse effects: Orally – nausea, vomiting, diarrhoea; possible photosensitivity with dermal use.

Interactions: None documented, although presence of coumarins may potentially trigger interactions with photosensitizing drugs and herbs when taken in therapeutic doses.

CRANBERRY
Vaccinium macrocarpon Herbal remedy.

Indications: Orally – for prevention and treatment of urinary tract infection, kidney stones, neurogenic bladder, diuretic, urinary deodorizer, blockage of urinary catheter, urostomy, stoma, wound healing. Also for type 2 diabetes mellitus, chronic fatigue syndrome, benign prostatic hyperplasia, common cold, influenza, poor memory, *Helicobacter pylori* infection.

Safety in pregnancy: Appears safe to use in pregnancy and breastfeeding. However, advise women to seek medical treatment for urinary tract infections, particularly if prone when not pregnant.

Contraindications and precautions: If consumed as preventative for urinary tract infection must be sugar-free to avoid exacerbating infections from sugar adhering to walls of ureters and bladder, increasing bacterial growth. Avoid with renal calculi – may increase stone formation in excessive or prolonged doses. Avoid in diabetes mellitus, especially juices that are high in sugar content. Avoid if aspirin allergy or asthma – large amounts could cause allergic reaction.

Adverse effects: Vulval or vaginal candida from prolonged use, especially if high sugar content, causing itching, irritation, increased frequency of micturition, nocturia. Stomach discomfort and diarrhoea with prolonged or excessive use. May increase risk of renal calculi and affect absorption of vitamin B12.

Interactions: Therapeutic oral doses, prolonged, excessive or inappropriate use may interact with anticoagulants and antiplatelet drugs: heparin, warfarin, aspirin, diclofenac, ibuprofen, enoxaparin. Also amitriptyline, diazepam. Anticoagulant herbs: angelica, clove, garlic, ginger, ginkgo, meadowsweet, Panax ginseng, poplar, red clover, turmeric.

CUMIN
Cuminum cyminum, Cuminum odorum Herbal remedy.

Indications: Orally – to stimulate menstruation. Also for flatulence, diarrhoea, abdominal colic, diuretic, stimulant, antispasmodic. Some cultures make cumin tea (jeera) for pregnancy wellbeing. Used in Ayurvedic medicine.

Safety in pregnancy: Appears safe in amounts commonly used in foods. Cumin tea safe in amounts up to one litre daily. AVOID THERAPEUTIC DOSES IN PRECONCEPTION PERIOD AND PREGNANCY unless under the supervision of a qualified medical herbalist or Ayurvedic practitioner. May contribute to miscarriage in first trimester in large amounts. May suppress testosterone levels in men, affecting fertility.

Contraindications and precautions: Avoid if allergic to cumin or other spices in the Apiaceae family. Avoid with diabetes mellitus, haemorrhagic and coagulation disorders, liver disease, renal disease; discontinue for at least two weeks prior to elective surgery. Do not consume more than one litre of cumin water or tea per day.

Adverse effects: Excessive or prolonged therapeutic doses may cause headache, nausea, dizziness, skin irritation, sweating, lowered blood sugar, renal or hepatic compromise. May be contaminated with fungi or bacteria or potentially harmful minerals.

Interactions: Therapeutic oral doses, prolonged, excessive or inappropriate use may interact with anticoagulants and antiplatelet drugs: heparin, warfarin, aspirin, diclofenac, ibuprofen, enoxaparin. Also antidiabetic medication. Anticoagulant herbs: angelica, clove, garlic, ginger, ginkgo, meadowsweet, Panax ginseng, poplar, red clover, turmeric. Hypoglycaemic herbs: devil's claw, fenugreek, Siberian ginseng.

CYPRESS
Cupressus sempervirens Herbal remedy.

Indications: Topically, essential oil in aromatherapy – for oedema, carpal tunnel syndrome, varicose veins, haemorrhoids, cystitis, wound healing, common cold, cough, bronchitis, as expectorant, relaxant, for pain relief, mood stimulant. Orally – for coughs, common colds, influenza, sore throat; benign prostatic hyperplasia.

Safety in pregnancy: Topically and by inhalation – essential oil in aromatherapy safe enough in pregnancy in doses up to 1.5% and up to 2% in labour and postnatally. Caution with oral therapeutic doses: insufficient information on safety in pregnancy or breastfeeding.

Contraindications and precautions: Topically, essential oil in aromatherapy – do not ingest. Do not use neat on skin or directly in a birthing pool. Do not apply directly to breasts in postnatal period, or wash with water before the baby starts feeding to avoid adverse neonatal effects from ingestion. Caution with hypertension – astringent properties may cause vasoconstriction. By inhalation – avoid with respiratory allergic conditions, for example asthma, hay fever. Use a diffuser for a maximum of 15–20 minutes in any hour; do not vaporize in the second stage of labour to avoid neonatal exposure; do not diffuse near neonates, elderly or ill people. Do not diffuse in public areas or use excessive amounts which spread to public areas of maternity unit, to avoid excessive exposure of the woman, baby, visitors, staff to potential adverse effects. Discontinue use if any allergic reactions occur to avoid accumulative reaction to specific chemicals – may lead to anaphylactic shock in severe cases. Store in a refrigerator to avoid rapid oxidation. Do not use with or store near homeopathic remedies. Orally – hypertension, renal disease; bleeding disorders. Discontinue at least two weeks prior to elective surgery.

Adverse effects: Topically, essential oil – skin irritation, especially if oil oxidized; avoid neat application. Orally – kidney irritation, respiratory allergic reactions.

Interactions: Therapeutic oral doses, prolonged, excessive or inappropriate use may interact with anticoagulants and antiplatelet drugs: heparin, warfarin, aspirin, diclofenac, ibuprofen, enoxaparin. Anticoagulant herbs: angelica, clove, garlic, ginger, ginkgo, meadowsweet, Panax ginseng, poplar, red clover, turmeric, willow bark.

DAGGA *see* **Cannabis**

DAGGER PLANT *see* Yucca

DAMIANA
Turnera diffusa, Turnera aphrodisiaca Herbal remedy.

Indications: Orally – for menopausal symptoms, premenstrual syndrome, fertility. Also for headache, mild depression, heartburn, constipation, asthma, enuresis, diabetes, sexual dysfunction, weight loss, to increase exercise performance, enhance cognitive function.

Safety in pregnancy: AVOID IN PRECONCEPTION PERIOD AND PREGNANCY – may be abortifacient. Caution: insufficient information available on safety in breastfeeding.

Contraindications and precautions: Avoid with diabetes mellitus.

Adverse effects: Large amounts taken orally reported to cause convulsions.

Interactions: Therapeutic oral doses, prolonged, excessive or inappropriate use may interact with diabetic medication. Hypoglycaemic herbs: chromium, devil's claw, fenugreek, garlic, horse chestnut, Panax ginseng, psyllium, Siberian ginseng.

DANDELION

Taraxacum officinale, Taraxacum vulgare Herbal remedy.

Indications: Orally – for oedema, heartburn, flatulence, constipation, anaemia, as a diuretic. Also for loss of appetite, gallstones, bile stimulation, joint and muscle pain, eczema, bruising, tonic, urinary tract infection.

Safety in pregnancy: Appears safe in amounts commonly used in foods. High in vitamins K and A; caution in pregnancy unless under the supervision of a medical herbalist.

Contraindications and precautions: Avoid with gallstones, stomach ulcers. Avoid if allergic to plants in the Asteraceae/Compositae plant family.

Adverse effects: Orally – stomach discomfort, diarrhoea, heartburn, allergic reactions, anaphylaxis. Topically – contact dermatitis, allergic reaction in those sensitive to chrysanthemums, marigolds, daisies, yarrow. May prolong bleeding time through inhibition of platelet aggregation, cause bruising.

Interactions: Therapeutic oral doses, prolonged, excessive or inappropriate use may interact with anticoagulants and antiplatelet drugs: heparin, warfarin, aspirin, diclofenac, ibuprofen, enoxaparin. Also antidiabetic medication; ondansetron, amitriptyline, theophylline, oestrogens, oral contraceptives, diuretics, lithium. Herbs: angelica, clove, devil's claw, fenugreek, garlic, ginger, ginkgo, meadowsweet, Panax ginseng, red clover, Siberian ginseng, turmeric, willow bark. Also oestrogenic herbs: black cohosh, blue cohosh, dong quai, evening primrose, fennel, fenugreek, ginkgo, ginseng, liquorice, raspberry leaf, red clover, vitex agnus castus.

DANGGUI *see* Angelica

DATE PALM

Phoenix dactylifera Herbal remedy.

Indications: Orally – fruit eaten as a popular means of initiating labour contractions to avoid induction. Therapeutic doses also used for respiratory symptoms, constipation. Pollen and flowers – for male infertility. Topically in cream form for ageing skin.

Safety in pregnancy: Considered a "forbidden fruit" in many Middle Eastern countries where date palms grow; said to have oestrogenic effects, possibly increasing risk of miscarriage. Question women about self-administration of herbal remedies to initiate labour and record in notes.

Contraindications and precautions: Avoid excessive consumption of fruit until 37 weeks' gestation – tannins and phytoestrogens may theoretically cause miscarriage or preterm labour. High in sugar – avoid with vaginal bacteriosis or candidiasis.

Do not confuse with edible palm oil (*Elaeis guineensis, Elaeis melanococca*) that comes from African palm and is safe in pregnancy.

Adverse effects: Allergic reactions from eating fruit in therapeutic doses and inhaling date palm pollen. Diarrhoea. Theoretically, disruption of uterine polarity at term from over-consumption.

Interactions: None documented, but in view of potential adverse effects, advice is to avoid concomitant use of oxytocic drugs and other herbal remedies intended to initiate labour – black cohosh, blue cohosh, castor oil, clary sage, evening primrose oil, raspberry leaf.

DEADLY NIGHTSHADE *see* Belladonna, herbal remedy, homeopathic remedy

DEERBERRY *see* Squaw vine and Wintergreen

DELPHINIUM *see* Staphysagria

DEVIL'S CLAW
Harpagophytum procumbens Herbal remedy.

Indications: Orally – to aid stalled labour, for menstrual problems. Also for allergic reactions, loss of appetite, backache, arthritis, gout, fibromyalgia, chest pain, indigestion, migraine, kidney and bladder disease. Topically – for skin injuries.

Safety in pregnancy: AVOID IN PREGNANCY unless under the supervision of a qualified medical herbalist – may have oxytocic effects, possibly causing miscarriage, preterm labour.

Contraindications and precautions: Orally – hypertension and hypotension, cardiac disease, diabetes mellitus, hyponatraemia, gallstones, peptic ulcer.

Adverse effects: Diarrhoea, allergic skin reactions, dysmenorrhoea, headache, tinnitus, loss of taste, hypertension, anxiety, dizziness, insomnia.

Interactions: Therapeutic oral doses, prolonged, excessive or inappropriate use may interact with diazepam, diclofenac, ibuprofen, amitriptyline, some anticoagulants. Anticoagulant herbs: angelica, clove, garlic, ginger, ginkgo, meadowsweet, Panax ginseng, poplar, red clover, turmeric.

DONG QUAI
Angelica sinensis Herbal remedy, also known as Chinese angelica.

Indications: Orally – popularly used in Chinese medicine for pregnancy-associated complications, dysmenorrhoea, premenstrual syndrome, menopausal symptoms, infertility. Also for migraine headache, constipation, osteoporosis, hypertension, rheumatoid arthritis, anaemia, allergic attacks, psoriasis, eczema. Topically – combined with other herbs in traditional Chinese remedy to treat premature ejaculation.

Safety in pregnancy: AVOID THERAPEUTIC ORAL DOSES IN PRECONCEPTION PERIOD AND IN PREGNANCY unless under the supervision of a qualified practitioner – has both stimulating and relaxing effects on uterine muscle; may affect embryonic development. Caution: insufficient information available on safety in breastfeeding – one report of neonatal hypertension, probably from maternal use.

Contraindications and precautions: Haemorrhagic disorders. Discontinue use at least two weeks prior to elective surgery. Hormone-sensitive disorders – endometriosis, uterine fibroids, breast, ovarian and uterine cancer. Systemic lupus erythematosus. Several other types of angelica are used in Japan and Korea – do not confuse with Angelica (*Angelica officinalis/Angelica archangelica*).

Adverse effects: Flatulence, burping, photosensitivity. Long-term therapeutic doses may be carcinogenic.

Interactions: Therapeutic oral doses, prolonged, excessive or inappropriate use may interact with anticoagulants and antiplatelet drugs: heparin, warfarin, aspirin, diclofenac, ibuprofen, enoxaparin. Also hormone replacement therapy, contraceptive Pill. Anticoagulant herbs: angelica, clove, garlic, ginger, ginkgo, meadowsweet, Panax ginseng, poplar, red clover, turmeric. Oestrogenic herbs: black cohosh, blue cohosh, dong quai, evening primrose, fennel, fenugreek, ginkgo, ginseng, liquorice, raspberry leaf, red clover, vitex agnus castus. Also possibly with black pepper.

ECHINACEA

Echinacea angustifolia, Echinacea purpura, Echinacea pallida Herbal remedy, also known as American cone flower.

Indications: Orally – for vaginal candidiasis. Primarily as immunostimulant, commonly used to prevent and treat the common cold; also for influenza, ear infection, urinary tract infection, herpes simplex virus, human papilloma virus, HIV/AIDS, septicaemia, tonsillitis, streptococcal infection, chronic fatigue syndrome, anxiety, migraine, heartburn, enhancing exercise performance. Topically – for gingivitis, abscess, skin wounds, ulcers, burns, eczema, psoriasis, ultraviolet radiation-induced skin damage, herpes simplex, thrush infection, bee stings, snake and mosquito bites, haemorrhoids.

Safety in pregnancy: Appears safe enough used in therapeutic doses orally or topically in the short term for five to seven days in pregnancy with no apparent adverse effects on the embryo/fetus. Caution: no information available on safety during breastfeeding.

Contraindications and precautions: Chemical constituents boost T-cell activity – avoid with autoimmune diseases, especially with gestational/pre-existing thyroid dysfunction; tendency to allergic reactions, intolerances, sensitivities. Do not use for children. Avoid with hepatic compromise including obstetric cholestasis. Do not confuse with Goldenseal.

Adverse effects: Nausea, vomiting, diarrhoea; unpleasant taste in mouth, dry, burning tongue; headache, allergic skin or respiratory reactions – may be severe. Rare cases of hepatic failure reported with prolonged use.

Interactions: Therapeutic oral doses, prolonged, excessive or inappropriate use may interact with caffeine, immunosuppressants; mild effect with warfarin. Herbs with possible effects on immune system: astralgus, elderberry, feverfew, turmeric.

ELDERBERRY
Sambucus nigra Herbal remedy.

Indications: Orally – for the common cold, influenza, chronic fatigue syndrome, allergic rhinitis, sciatica, headache, toothache, as a diuretic, laxative, to stimulate immune function. Topically – as an oral mouthwash for gingivitis.

Safety in pregnancy: Appears safe in amounts commonly found in cooked foods. Caution: insufficient information on safety in pregnancy, breastfeeding.

Contraindications and precautions: Do not consume raw leaves, unripe or uncooked berries – they contain a potentially toxic cyanide-producing chemical; cooking eliminates the toxin. Avoid with autoimmune diseases.

Adverse effects: Raw, unripe fruit, seeds, leaves cause nausea, vomiting, diarrhoea, weakness, dizziness, numbness. Pollen and some commercially produced extracts may cause allergic reaction, including dyspnoea, rhinitis.

Interactions: Therapeutic oral doses, prolonged, excessive or inappropriate use may interact with fluoxetine, ondansetron, propranolol, glucocorticoids, immunosuppressants, possibly decongestants and some antibiotics. Herbs: berberis, ginger, liquorice.

ELEPHANT DUNG
Traditional remedy used in southern Africa, also known as Ndove yenzou.

Indications: Orally – crushed, added to water, drunk during third trimester to aid childbirth, ease placental delivery, prevent perineal lacerations, boost immune system. Also inhaled as smoke from burning dung, as an analgesic for headache, toothache, to clear sinus congestion, for epistaxis.

Safety in pregnancy: Caution: no information available on safety. Contains very little bacteria, therefore relatively sterile; consists of semi-digested leaves, often used in isolation as traditional remedies. Chemical constituents and therapeutic effects depend on elephant diet – wide geographical variations.

Contraindications and precautions: In some areas may contain ingested hallucinogenic mushroom.

Adverse effects: None documented, but given potential chemical effects of plants contained within, advice is to remain alert to apparently idiopathic physiological symptoms.

Interactions: None documented.

ELEUTHERO *see* Siberian ginseng

EPHEDRA *see* Ma huang

ERGOT

Claviceps purpurea Herbal remedy sometimes called *Secale cereale* due to rye on which ergot grows.

Indications: Orally – for menorrhagia, metrorrhagia, to shorten third stage of labour, postpartum haemorrhage, atonic uterus.

Safety in pregnancy: AVOID ORAL USE IN PREGNANCY, LABOUR AND POSTPARTUM PERIOD – in its original plant form, herbal ergot is toxic and may interfere with pregnancy and birth physiology, hypertension and other conditions.

Contraindications and precautions: Major risk in women with cardiac, hepatic, renal or vascular disease. Do not confuse with pharmaceutical preparations of ergometrine. Do not confuse with Secale, homeopathic remedy.

Adverse effects: Orally, usually after repeated doses – nausea, vomiting, diarrhoea, abdominal pain, muscle weakness and pain, numbness and tingling of fingers and toes, extreme thirst, coldness, itching skin, tachycardia, hypotension, shock, confusion, convulsions, cyanosis, unconsciousness, death.

Interactions: Therapeutic oral doses, prolonged, excessive or inappropriate use may interact with antidepressants, monoamine oxidase inhibitors, bromocriptine, pentazocine, epinephrine, antihypertensives. Herbs: bitter orange, caffeine, country mallow, ephedra, Hawaiian baby woodrose, St John's wort.

EUCALYPTUS

Eucalyptus globulus, Eucalyptus smithii, Eucalyptus odorata Herbal remedy, also known as Blue gum.

Indications: Orally – for pyrexia, heartburn, respiratory tract infections, whooping cough, asthma, pulmonary tuberculosis, acne, wound care, burns, ringworm, bleeding gums, neuralgia. Essential oil, orally – for respiratory tract infection, sinusitis, asthma. Topically and by inhalation, essential oil also used for rheumatic complaints, arthritis, genital herpes, head lice, as insect repellent, as anti-inflammatory, muscular analgesic, to increase alertness, reduce pyrexia.

Safety in pregnancy: Appears safe in amounts commonly used in foods. Essential oil used in aromatherapy is safe in doses up to 1.5% in pregnancy and 2% in labour and postnatal period.

Contraindications and precautions: Orally – avoid eucalyptus leaf in diabetes mellitus, may cause hypoglycaemia. Essential oil, topically or by inhalation – avoid with asthma, may trigger attack. Do not ingest and keep out of reach of children – several Australian reports of neurotoxicity in infants/children exposed to neat dermal essential oil or oral ingestion. Do not use neat on skin or directly in a birthing pool. Do not apply directly to breasts in postnatal period, or wash with water before the baby starts feeding to avoid adverse neonatal effects from ingestion. Use a diffuser for a maximum of 15–20 minutes in any hour; do not vaporize in the second stage of labour to avoid neonatal exposure. Do not diffuse near neonates, elderly or ill people. Do not diffuse near cats – toxic. Do not diffuse in public areas or use excessive amounts which spread to public areas of maternity unit, to avoid excessive exposure of the woman, baby, visitors and staff to potential adverse effects. Discontinue use if any allergic reactions occur to avoid accumulative reaction to specific chemicals – may lead to anaphylactic shock in severe cases. Store in a refrigerator to avoid rapid oxidation. Do not use with or store near homeopathic remedies. There are several types of eucalyptus, most considered safe in pregnancy, labour and postnatally, but caution with other types; for example *Eucalyptus citriodora* (lemon-scented) is considered safe, but *Eucalyptus camphora* contains higher proportions of camphor, and is therefore contraindicated. Keep all types of eucalyptus away from domestic cats and do not vaporize if cats are nearby – can cause unstable gait, drooling, ill health.

Adverse effects: Orally – nausea, vomiting, diarrhoea. Ingestion of more than one millilitre of essential oil (adult) can cause epigastric pain, muscle weakness, shallow respiration, rapid pulse, apnoea, slurred speech, clammy skin, central nervous system depression, pinpoint pupils, coma, death. Essential oil – topically or by inhalation, excessive or prolonged exposure can lead to agitation, drowsiness, ataxia, muscle weakness, convulsions; risk of toxicity is greater in children and babies. Contact dermatitis can occur from skin contact with pollen, leaves or oil due to eucalyptol constituent. Toxicity can also occur from prolonged inhalation of oil, such as in diffusers. Those allergic to tea tree should avoid eucalyptus – similar chemical constituents.

Interactions: Therapeutic oral doses, prolonged, excessive or inappropriate use may interact with amphetamines, antidiabetic medication, ondansetron, propranolol, theophylline, verapamil, diazepam, non-steroidal anti-inflammatories, warfarin, amitriptyline. Hepatotoxic herbs: borage, butterbur, coltsfoot, comfrey, forget-me-not, golden ragwort, groundsel, hemp agrimony, hound's tongue, tansy ragwort. Hypoglycaemic herbs: bitter melon, chromium, devil's claw, fenugreek, garlic, guar gum, horse chestnut, Panax ginseng, prickly pear cactus, psyllium, Siberian ginseng.

EUPHORBIA

Chamaesyce hirta, Euphorbia hirta Herbal remedy, also known as Asthma plant, Snakeweed.

Indications: Orally – for asthma, bronchitis, catarrh, hay fever, as an expectorant. Used in Ayurvedic medicine as an emetic; also for worms, dysentery, gonorrhoea, digestive problems.

Safety in pregnancy: AVOID IN PREGNANCY AND BREASTFEEDING – may cause smooth muscle contraction leading to miscarriage, preterm labour, hypertonic uterine action.

Contraindications and precautions: Gastrointestinal conditions. Avoid skin contact with fresh herb. Do not confuse with *Euphrasia officinale* (eyebright).

Adverse effects: Contact dermatitis, eye irritation, gastrointestinal inflammation.

Interactions: None documented.

EUROPEAN BARBERRY *see* Barberry

EVENING PRIMROSE OIL

Oenothera biennis Herbal remedy, often available in commercially produced oil capsules or other forms.

Indications: Orally – to prevent pre-eclampsia, induce or accelerate labour, for premenstrual syndrome, mastalgia including breast engorgement, to increase lactation, for polycystic ovary syndrome, endometriosis, menopausal symptoms. Also for skin disorders, rheumatoid arthritis, osteoporosis, Raynaud's syndrome, multiple sclerosis, dry eyes; liver conditions, hypercholesterolaemia, chronic fatigue syndrome, attention deficit-hyperactivity disorder, obesity, ulcerative colitis, irritable bowel syndrome, peptic ulcer. Topically – for various skin conditions.

Safety in pregnancy: Appears safe enough towards term in therapeutic doses when taken under the supervision of a midwife, doctor or qualified medical herbalist. Thought to aid cervical ripening, but preterm or excessive doses may disrupt uterine polarity, causing prolonged rather than shortened labour, delay in membrane rupture, poor descent of presenting part, increased need for oxytocin supplementation, potentially increased need for operative delivery, especially in primigravidae. Inconclusive evidence for professional use for post-dates pregnancy, with no consensus on dosage. Question women about self-administration of herbal remedies to initiate labour and record in notes. Considerable incorrect and potentially harmful online information advocating use for post-dates pregnancy, often in conjunction with other herbs – advise caution. Appears safe when breastfeeding.

Contraindications and precautions: Epilepsy (controversial, but advice is to avoid in pregnancy), schizophrenia. Do not use in conjunction with other herbal or medicinal methods of cervical ripening or to stimulate contractions, for example Raspberry leaf, Clary sage, Castor oil, Black cohosh, Blue cohosh or pharmaceutical oxytocic drugs. May prolong bleeding times: discontinue at least two weeks before surgery; do not use with antepartum haemorrhage, retained products of conception, excessive lochial discharges, haemorrhagic disorders.

Adverse effects: Orally – gastrointestinal symptoms, headache, dizziness, bruising, bleeding. May trigger epileptiform fits, although evidence is inconclusive; risk is likely to be related to interactions with medication in those with known epilepsy.

Interactions: Therapeutic oral doses, prolonged, excessive or inappropriate use may interact with lithium, phenothiazines, anaesthetics. Also anticoagulants and antiplatelet drugs: heparin, warfarin, aspirin, diclofenac, ibuprofen, enoxaparin. Anticoagulant herbs: angelica, clove, garlic, ginger, ginkgo, meadowsweet, Panax ginseng, poplar, red clover, turmeric.

FALSE JASMINE *see* **Gelsemium, herbal remedy**

FALSE UNICORN ROOT
Chamaelirium luteum Herbal remedy.

Indications: Orally – for threatened miscarriage, gestational sickness, to normalize hormones after oral contraceptive use, ovarian cysts, menstrual problems, menopausal symptoms. Traditionally, root used for gynaecological conditions and infertility. Also as a diuretic, for digestive problems, intestinal worms.

Safety in pregnancy: AVOID IN PRECONCEPTION PERIOD AND PREGNANCY, unless under the supervision of a qualified medical herbalist: potential uterine stimulant. Thought to be safe in labour and breastfeeding but advise caution: some authorities regard it as unsafe throughout the childbearing year.

Contraindications and precautions: Gastrointestinal inflammatory conditions.

Adverse effects: Nausea and vomiting in large doses.

Interactions: Therapeutic oral doses, prolonged, excessive or inappropriate use may interact with amitriptyline, clozapine, codeine, fentanyl, fluoxetine, methadone, ondansetron, lithium. Herbs – none documented, but in view of possible effects, advise caution with oestrogenic herbs: black cohosh, blue cohosh, dong quai, evening primrose, fennel, fenugreek, ginkgo, ginseng, liquorice, raspberry leaf, red clover, vitex agnus castus.

FENNEL
Foeniculum vulgare Herbal remedy, also known as Sweet fennel.

Indications: Orally – to facilitate labour, increase lactation, to promote menstruation, for dysmenorrhoea, reduced libido, as a tea for infant colic. Also for coughs, bronchitis, backache, enuresis, heartburn, flatulence, colitis, nausea, constipation, loss of appetite, anxiety, arthritis, cancer, diabetes, insomnia, vaginal atrophy, sunburn. Topically – essential oil for wound healing, as an antispasmodic, particularly for intestinal cramps and inflammatory bowel conditions, analgesic, antioxidant, antibacterial.

Safety in pregnancy: Consumption of vegetable or seeds appears safe in amounts commonly used in foods. AVOID THERAPEUTIC ORAL DOSES AND TOPICAL OR INHALATIONAL USE OF ESSENTIAL OIL IN PREGNANCY – phytoestrogens may cause miscarriage, preterm labour; caution in labour – risk of hypertonic uterine action. Avoid consumption of large amounts of fennel tea in pregnancy. Minimal amounts of tea may be safe enough in babies to ease abdominal colic; large amounts may lead to neurotoxicity.

Contraindications and precautions: Avoid therapeutic oral doses or excessive consumption of vegetable with haemorrhagic disorders. Essential oil, topically or by inhalation – do not use if menstruating or with hormone-sensitive conditions – breast, uterine and ovarian cancer, endometriosis, uterine fibroids. Keep out of reach of children; do not use for babies. Do not ingest. Do not use neat on skin or directly in a birthing pool. Do not apply directly to breasts in postnatal period, or wash with water before the baby starts feeding to avoid adverse neonatal effects from ingestion. The advice is not to diffuse in the postnatal period, particularly near neonates, elderly or ill people; if used, for a maximum of 15–20 minutes in any hour. Discontinue use if any allergic reactions occur to avoid accumulative reaction to specific chemicals – may lead to anaphylactic shock in severe cases. Do not use with or store near homeopathic remedies.

Adverse effects: Orally – ingestion of herbal remedy or excessive consumption of vegetable in diet may cause bleeding, bruising, especially in those with haemorrhagic disorders or on prophylactic anticoagulant therapy. Topically, essential oil – allergic reactions, gastrointestinal discomfort, photosensitivity, skin irritation. There have been reports of fits occurring from ingestion of essential oil.

Interactions: Therapeutic oral doses, prolonged, excessive or inappropriate use may interact with anticoagulants and antiplatelet drugs: heparin, warfarin, aspirin, diclofenac, ibuprofen, enoxaparin. Also certain strong antibiotics, contraceptive Pill, calcium channel blockers, antifungals, fentanyl, lignocaine, hormone replacement therapy, tamoxifen. Anticoagulant herbs: angelica, clove, garlic, ginger, ginkgo, meadowsweet, Panax ginseng, poplar, red clover, turmeric. Oestrogenic herbs: black cohosh, blue cohosh, dong quai, evening primrose, fennel, fenugreek, ginkgo, ginseng, liquorice, raspberry leaf, red clover, vitex agnus castus.

FENUGREEK

Trigonella foenum-graecum Herbal remedy.

Indications: Orally – to stimulate lactation, for dysmenorrhoea, polycystic ovary syndrome, menopausal symptoms; to increase libido, for male infertility, impotence. Also for loss of appetite, heartburn, oesophageal reflux, gastritis, constipation, obesity, kidney disease, mouth ulcers, bronchitis, coughs, baldness, exercise performance. Topically – for localized inflammation, muscle pain, wounds, eczema.

Safety in pregnancy: Appears safe in amounts commonly used in foods. AVOID THERAPEUTIC ORAL DOSES IN PRECONCEPTION PERIOD AND PREGNANCY – possible oxytocic and uterine-stimulating effects. Several case reports of hydrocephalus, anencephaly, cleft palate, spina bifida in babies of women taking it in pregnancy, and of babies born with unusual body odour similar to maple syrup urine disease. Considered safe for short-term maternal use to aid lactation, either as tea or in powder form – possibly increases prolactin levels, although evidence is inconclusive and contradictory. No apparent long-term effects.

Contraindications and precautions: Haemorrhagic or coagulation disorders, diabetes mellitus. If the neonate has unusual body odour, do not confuse with maple syrup urine disease. Consider maternal fenugreek consumption if the baby is born with maple syrup-like odour. Do not use for babies.

Adverse effects: Orally, topically and by inhalation – allergic reactions including diarrhoea, heartburn, abdominal distension, nausea, flatulence, dizziness, headaches; large amounts of powdered form may cause hypoglycaemia, shock.

Interactions: Therapeutic oral doses, prolonged, excessive or inappropriate use may interact with anticoagulants and antiplatelet drugs: heparin, warfarin, aspirin, diclofenac, ibuprofen, enoxaparin. Also antidiabetic medication, theophylline. Anticoagulant herbs: angelica, clove, garlic, ginger, ginkgo, red clover, turmeric, willow bark. Hypoglycaemic herbs: devil's claw, Panax ginseng, Siberian ginseng. May cause allergic reactions in those sensitive to plants in the Fabaceae family including peanuts, soybeans, chickpeas, green peas.

FEVERFEW

Tanacetum parthenium, Chrysanthemum parthenium Herbal remedy.

Indications: Orally – for miscarriage, menstrual problems, infertility. Also primarily for headache and migraine; for pyrexia, arthritis, psoriasis, allergies, asthma, nausea and vomiting, anaemia, common cold, earache, muscular tension, oedema, diarrhoea, indigestion, flatulence. Topically – for toothache, general stimulant, intestinal parasites.

Safety in pregnancy: AVOID ORAL USE IN PREGNANCY – may cause threatened miscarriage, preterm labour. Caution: little information on safety during breastfeeding or with topical use.

Contraindications and precautions: Avoid with haemorrhagic/coagulation disorders. Avoid if sensitive to plants in the Asteraceae/Compositae family – ragweed, chrysanthemums, marigolds, daisies.

Adverse effects: Allergic reactions; chewing fresh leaves can cause oral and lip inflammation, mouth ulcers, loss of sense of taste.

Interactions: Therapeutic oral doses, prolonged, excessive or inappropriate use may interact with anticoagulants and antiplatelet drugs: heparin, warfarin, aspirin, diclofenac, ibuprofen, enoxaparin. Also amitriptyline, ondansetron, propranolol, theophylline, verapamil, diazepam, chlorpromazine, tamoxifen, non-steroidal anti-inflammatories. Anticoagulant herbs: angelica, clove, garlic, ginger, ginkgo, meadowsweet, Panax ginseng, poplar, red clover, turmeric, willow bark.

FLAXSEED
Linum usitatissimum Herbal remedy, also known as Linseed.

Indications: Orally – for menopausal symptoms, mastalgia. Primarily for constipation, diarrhoea, irritable bowel syndrome, ulcerative colitis. Also for diabetes mellitus, hypercholesterolaemia, hypertension, weight loss, depression, cystitis, coughs, rheumatoid arthritis, nephritis, various cancers. Topically – for burns, acne, eczema, psoriasis, skin inflammation.

Safety in pregnancy: Appears safe in amounts commonly used in foods. AVOID THERAPEUTIC ORAL DOSES IN PREGNANCY – may have oestrogenic effects, possibly causing miscarriage, preterm labour. Appears safe enough in small doses during breastfeeding – observe neonates for diarrhoea.

Contraindications and precautions: Caution with general use in pregnancy; discontinue if any excess uterine action occurs, possibly due to severe diarrhoea. Do not consume raw or unripe flaxseed – contain cyanide-like chemicals but cooking appears to negate this. Increased risk of bleeding – avoid in haemorrhagic conditions, antepartum haemorrhage, prior to elective surgery, heavy postnatal lochia. Avoid in diabetes mellitus, inflammatory bowel disease, hormone-sensitive conditions, hypertension, hypotension.

Adverse effects: Diarrhoea, allergic and anaphylactic reactions. May lower serum glucose levels.

Interactions: Therapeutic oral doses, prolonged, excessive or inappropriate use may interact with anticoagulants, antiplatelet drugs: heparin, warfarin, aspirin, diclofenac, ibuprofen, enoxaparin. Also antidiabetic medication, certain antibiotics, antihypertensives, oral contraceptives, hormone replacement therapy, diuretics, other drugs taken orally immediately prior to flaxseed ingestion due to poor absorption. Anticoagulant herbs: angelica, clove, garlic, ginger, ginkgo,

Panax ginseng. Hypoglycaemic herbs: bitter melon, chromium, devil's claw, fenugreek, garlic, guar gum, horse chestnut, psyllium, Siberian ginseng. Hypotensive herbs: coenzyme Q10, devil's claw, fish oil, stinging nettle. Oestrogenic herbs: black cohosh, blue cohosh, dong quai, evening primrose, fennel, fenugreek, ginkgo, ginseng, liquorice, raspberry leaf, red clover, vitex agnus castus.

FRANKINCENSE

Boswellia carteri Herbal remedy, also known as Olibanum.

Indications: Topically and by inhalation, essential oil in aromatherapy – as a sedative, antiseptic, antibacterial, decongestant, expectorant. Useful for anxiety, fear, hysteria, transition stage of labour, postnatal "blues"; constipation, abdominal colic, flatulence; pain relief for pregnancy aches, labour pain, postnatal recovery; sinus congestion, cough, common cold. Orally – for colic, flatulence, general wellbeing. Popular in Ayurvedic medicine.

Safety in pregnancy: Essential oil used in aromatherapy appears safe in doses up to 1.5% in pregnancy and 2% in labour and postnatal period. There is some controversy on safety due to ketone content (emmenagoguic) but these are trace elements; most authorities suggest oil is safe in small amounts. Orally – little information available on safety – advise caution unless under the supervision of an appropriately qualified practitioner.

Contraindications and precautions: Essential oil – do not ingest. Do not use neat on skin or directly in a birthing pool. Use a diffuser for a maximum of 15–20 minutes in any hour; do not vaporize in the second stage of labour to avoid neonatal exposure; do not diffuse near neonates, elderly or ill people. Do not diffuse in public areas or use excessive amounts which spread to public areas of maternity unit, to avoid excessive exposure of the woman, baby, visitors and staff to potential adverse effects. Discontinue use if any allergic reactions occur to avoid accumulative reaction to specific chemicals – may lead to anaphylactic shock in severe cases. Store in a refrigerator; do not use with or store near homeopathic remedies. Caution with disposal of unused essential oil blends containing frankincense: has prolonged toxic effect on aquatic life, so do not dispose in sources of fresh water, for example lakes. Orally – avoid with antenatal, postnatal haemorrhage, coagulation or haemorrhagic disorders.

Adverse effects: Topically – skin irritation, especially if oil has oxidized: avoid out-of-date oils. Orally – nausea, vomiting, heartburn, acid reflux.

Interactions: Therapeutic oral doses, prolonged, excessive or inappropriate use may interact with anticoagulants: heparin, warfarin, enoxaparin; antiplatelet drugs: aspirin; anti-inflammatories: diclofenac, ibuprofen. Also cholesterol-lowering drugs. Herbs: none documented, but caution with anticoagulant herbs: angelica, clove, garlic, ginger, ginkgo, meadowsweet, Panax ginseng, turmeric, willow bark.

GARLIC

Allium sativum Herbal remedy.

Indications: Orally – for pre-eclampsia, vaginal candidiasis, vaginal trichomoniasis, menstrual disorders. Also for hypertension, hypotension, hyperlipidaemia, obesity, chronic fatigue syndrome, *Helicobacter pylori* infection, to prevent and treat various cancers, for bacterial and fungal infections, ringworm. Topically – oil used for alopecia, candidiasis, athlete's foot, verrucae, warts, corns.

Safety in pregnancy: Appears safe in amounts commonly used in foods. AVOID THERAPEUTIC ORAL DOSES (SUPPLEMENTS) IN PREGNANCY – may be abortifacient in large doses, although this is unconfirmed. Excessive consumption in late pregnancy may affect aroma of amniotic fluid and flavour/aroma of breast milk.

Contraindications and precautions: Avoid therapeutic oral doses (supplements) with threatened miscarriage, antepartum haemorrhage, excessive postnatal lochia, retained products of conception, haemorrhagic disorders, due to anticoagulant effects of allicin content; discontinue prior to surgery. Avoid with hypotension, diabetes mellitus.

Adverse effects: Malodorous breath, body odour, nausea, vomiting, belching, flatulence, diarrhoea, weight loss, dizziness, insomnia, allergic reactions; increased risk of bleeding with excessive use.

Interactions: Therapeutic oral doses, prolonged, excessive or inappropriate use may interact with anticoagulants and antiplatelet drugs: heparin, warfarin, aspirin, diclofenac, ibuprofen, enoxaparin. Also antidiabetic medication, certain anaesthetic drugs, isoniazid. Anticoagulant herbs: angelica, clove, ginger, ginkgo, red clover, turmeric, vitamin E, willow. Hypoglycaemic herbs: devil's claw, fenugreek, Panax ginseng, Siberian ginseng. Hypotensive herbs: cat's claw, coenzyme Q10, stinging nettle. Also eicosapentaenoic acid (EPA), fish oil – may enhance antithrombotic effects.

GEGEN *see* Kudzu

GELSEMIUM

Gelsemium sempiverens Herbal remedy, also known as Yellow jasmine, False jasmine.

Indications: Orally – traditionally used in Ayurvedic medicine as an analgesic for trigeminal neuralgia and migraine headaches, asthma and respiratory conditions.

Safety in pregnancy: AVOID ORAL USE IN PREGNANCY – all parts of the plant are highly toxic.

Contraindications and precautions: Avoid unless under the supervision of an appropriately qualified practitioner. Do not confuse with Gelsemium, homeopathic remedy.

Adverse effects: Headache, double vision, dysphagia, dizziness, muscle weakness or rigidity, convulsions, dyspnoea, bradycardia. Death due to failure of respiratory muscles can occasionally occur.

Interactions: None documented.

GELSEMIUM

Gelsemium sempiverens Homeopathic remedy from Yellow jasmine.

Obstetric indications: Influenza-like symptoms: dull, heavy headache, flushed face; trembling, shivers; weakness, poor muscle coordination; dull, heavy, painful backache and cold sensation along spine; lack of thirst. Yellow discharge, for example coated tongue. Profuse urination. Labour – anticipatory anxiety, distressing back pain, exhaustion, even at start. Contractions distressing, weak, cease on vaginal examination; labour may progress after urination.

Key features: Exhaustion and weariness with heavy eyelids, heavy feeling. Slow onset of condition. No sweating, not thirsty, trembling.

Emotional symptoms: Apathy, indifference, lack of willpower. Wants to be left alone, but fears being alone; dreads the birth; fears losing control. Cannot focus thoughts; answers slowly.

Better for: Urination; bending forwards; sweating; stimulants.

Worse for: Damp, warm weather; during thunderstorm; morning; when thinking about ailment; emotion; excitement; bad news.

Safety: Do not use if there are any medical or obstetric complications. Not to be used as a replacement for standard medical care. Do not use with aromatherapy essential oils, topically or by inhalation, or with antacids, decongestants, laxatives or cough lozenges – inactivates the remedy. Do not take with food or drink. Do not take prophylactically – may lead to reverse proving. Should not be used by women who do not fit the symptom picture to avoid reverse proving. To be handled by the intended recipient only. Do not confuse with Gelsemium, herbal remedy. Do not confuse with Jasmine, herbal remedy.

GENTIAN

Gentiana lutea, Gentiana acaulis Herbal remedy.

Indications: Orally – to stimulate menstruation, for sinusitis, loss of appetite, flatulence, diarrhoea, heartburn, vomiting; fever, hysteria, hypertension, diabetes mellitus, as an antispasmodic, antiseptic. Topically – for wounds, cancer. Also, available as liquid Bach Flower Remedy taken orally, diluted in spring water, for doubt and negative outlook.

Safety in pregnancy: Oral use generally appears safe; no real evidence on safety in pregnancy. Bach Flower Remedy appears safe.

Contraindications and precautions: Hypotension. Do not confuse with Gentian, homeopathic remedy. Do not confuse with white hellebore (*Veratrum album*) – flowering plant can be incorrectly identified as gentian. Do not confuse with gentian violet, topical antiseptic dye formerly used to treat fungal skin disorders, now banned in the USA and Canada, both for humans and animals, due to fears over toxicity and high iodine levels. Avoid Bach Flower Remedy with liver disease, alcohol dependency, severe mental health issues.

Adverse effects: Orally, sometimes in combination with other herbs – gastrointestinal disturbance, allergic skin reactions. No known adverse effects from topical use, although skin reactions possible in susceptible women.

Interactions: Therapeutic oral doses, prolonged, excessive or inappropriate use may interact with antihypertensives and hypotensive herbs: cat's claw, coenzyme Q10, fish oil, stinging nettle.

GENTIAN

Gentiana lutea Homeopathic remedy from yellow gentian.

Obstetric indications: Influenza; headaches; fear. Labour contractions distressing, weak, pass up the back and extend to the hips, cease during vaginal examination. Pain – sharp; stitching; spasmodic; sensation as if the uterus is being squeezed.

Key features: Influenza-like symptoms: trembling, heavy limbs, weakness, lack of coordination, shivering with cold sensation along spine. Lack of thirst, headache, dull backache, drooping eyelids, flushed face, coated tongue, profuse urination.

Emotional symptoms: Apathetic, indifferent, wants to be alone yet fears being alone. Dreads the birth, fears losing control. Cannot grasp thoughts, answers slowly, lacks willpower.

Better for: Urination; bending forwards; sweating; stimulants.

Worse for: Damp, warm weather; thunderstorms; afternoon; when thinking about ailment or situation; emotion; receiving bad news.

Safety: Do not use if there are any medical or obstetric complications. Not to be used as a replacement for standard medical care. Do not use with aromatherapy essential oils, topically or by inhalation, or with antacids, decongestants, laxatives or cough lozenges – inactivates the remedy. Do not take with food or drink. Do not take prophylactically – may lead to reverse proving. Should not be used by women who do not fit the symptom picture to avoid reverse proving. To be handled by the intended recipient only. Do not confuse with Gentian, herbal remedy.

GERANIUM

Pelargonium graveolens Herbal remedy, sometimes known as Rose geranium.

Indications: Topically – essential oil used in aromatherapy for backache, labour pain, postnatal recovery, anxiety, mood swings, skin conditions, wound healing, antibacterial, antifungal, anti-inflammatory, astringent, diuretic. As compress, leaves used for oedema, breast engorgement. By inhalation – essential oil used for relaxation, to uplift mood, deodorize environment. Orally, as a tea – for the common cold, neuropathic pain, diarrhoea, depression, weight loss, to improve athletic performance. Popular in Ayurvedic medicine.

Safety in pregnancy: Essential oil, topically or by inhalation in aromatherapy – appears safe in doses up to 1.5% in pregnancy and 2% in labour and postnatal period. AVOID THERAPEUTIC ORAL DOSES IN PREGNANCY unless under the supervision of an appropriately qualified practitioner.

Contraindications and precautions: Essential oil, topically and by inhalation – caution with hypertensive women as astringent effect may cause vasoconstriction. Beware effect on women prone to hay fever and asthma triggered by flower pollen – possible psychosomatic effect. Contains chemicals which may lift mood and others that may depress mood – effects may vary between individuals, but advise caution with women with mental health issues. Avoid if known allergy to geraniol (monoterpinoid alcohol) or perfumes containing geranium. Do not ingest. Do not use neat on skin or directly in a birthing pool. Use a diffuser for a maximum of 15–20 minutes in any hour; do not vaporize in the second stage of labour to avoid neonatal exposure. Not suitable for babies and infants; do not diffuse near neonates, elderly or ill people. Do not diffuse in public areas or use excessive amounts which spread to public areas of maternity unit, to avoid excessive exposure of the woman, baby, visitors and staff to potential adverse effects. Do not apply directly to breasts in postnatal period, or wash with water before the baby starts feeding to avoid adverse neonatal effects from ingestion. Discontinue use if any allergic reactions occur to avoid accumulative reaction to specific chemicals – may lead to anaphylactic shock in severe cases. Do not use with or store near homeopathic remedies. Good quality geranium oil is expensive – may be adulterated with cheaper, similar-smelling oils, so purchase from reputable suppliers. Store in a refrigerator to avoid rapid oxidation. Do not confuse with East Indian or Turkish geranium oil (known as palmarosa). Orally – avoid with autoimmune diseases; psoriasis, rheumatoid arthritis, systemic lupus erythematosus; may activate antibodies that trigger autoimmune responses. Toxic for dogs – do not allow them to eat leaves.

Adverse effects: Topically, essential oil in aromatherapy – dermatitis, burning sensation, light-headedness, nausea, headache, eye irritation – probably due to geraniol content. Women with hay fever triggered by flower pollen may experience psychosomatic effect from inhalation of essential oil vapours.

Interactions: Therapeutic oral doses, prolonged, excessive or inappropriate use may theoretically interact with anticoagulants, antidiabetic medication and herbs.

GINGER
Zingiber officinale Herbal remedy.

Indications: Orally – popularly used for nausea and vomiting, including pregnancy sickness. Also for colic, diarrhoea, heartburn, flatulence, irritable bowel syndrome, loss of appetite; dysmenorrhoea, menorrhagia, migraine headache, anorexia, respiratory tract infections. Topically – essential oil used in aromatherapy as analgesic, mood, circulatory and digestive stimulant, to prevent ageing, for hair and scalp health. Used in Chinese and Ayurvedic medicine.

Safety in pregnancy: Appears safe in amounts commonly used in foods. Orally, for pregnancy sickness – some suggestion of increased risk of stillbirth or adverse effect on fetal sex hormones (inconclusive evidence). AVOID ESSENTIAL OIL TOPICALLY OR ORALLY IN PREGNANCY – thought to stimulate uterine contractions, causing miscarriage, preterm labour, hypertonic uterine action; can be used with caution in labour, in doses up to 2%. Caution in early postnatal period, maximum dose 2%, but avoid with excessive lochial bleeding, retained products of conception.

Contraindications and precautions: Orally – appears safe in pregnancy in amounts commonly found in foods. Therapeutic oral doses – fresh ginger root, usually in tea form, is safer than dried ginger; must be common ginger, *Zingiber officinale*. Controversy over safe maximum daily dose – UK advises maximum 1g grated raw root ginger (half a teaspoon), USA advises 2g (5ml teaspoon); Norway advises against use of all commercially prepared ginger supplements. Note: Biscuits do not contain therapeutic doses of ginger, and their high sugar content causes peaks and troughs of blood sugar that may exacerbate nausea – do not advise ginger biscuits for pregnancy sickness. Also discourage ginger products containing high levels of sugar, for example lollipops, crystallized ginger. Avoid ginger completely if there is a history of repeated miscarriage; discontinue use with threatened miscarriage or antepartum haemorrhage; avoid with haemorrhagic/coagulation disorders or for women on anticoagulants/drugs or herbs with similar action. Check clotting factors if woman has used therapeutic doses of ginger for more than three weeks. Admission with threatened miscarriage or antepartum haemorrhage – check if the woman has self-administered ginger in therapeutic doses continuously for a prolonged time. Discontinue at least two weeks prior to surgery. Avoid with diabetes mellitus – may affect blood sugar levels. Not suitable for treatment if nausea, vomiting accompanied by heartburn. Do not confuse with Chinese ginger (Alpinia), wild ginger (Asarabacca), wall ginger (common stonecrop), green ginger (wormwood). Essential oil, topically in labour or postnatal period – do not ingest. Do not use neat on skin or directly in a birthing pool. Do not apply directly to breasts in postnatal period, or wash with water before the baby starts feeding to avoid adverse neonatal effects from ingestion. Use a diffuser for a maximum of 15–20 minutes in any hour; do not vaporize in the second stage of labour to avoid neonatal exposure; do not diffuse near neonates, elderly or ill people. Do not diffuse in public areas or use excessive amounts which spread to public areas of maternity unit, to avoid excessive exposure of the woman, baby, visitors and staff to potential adverse effects. Not to be used by pregnant staff caring for labouring women. Discontinue use if any allergic reactions occur to avoid accumulative reaction to specific chemicals – may lead to anaphylactic shock in severe cases. Store in a refrigerator; do not use with or store near homeopathic remedies.

Adverse effects: Prolonged use of therapeutic doses (continuous daily use for more than three weeks) may cause bruising, vaginal bleeding or spotting due to strong anticoagulant effect. May cause abdominal discomfort, heartburn, diarrhoea, irritation in mouth and throat, skin irritation. May increase insulin levels, causing hypoglycaemia in diabetic women. Topically, essential oil – contact dermatitis. May interfere with results of clotting factor tests, increasing bleeding time.

Interactions: Therapeutic oral doses, prolonged, excessive or inappropriate use, including prolonged consumption of ginger tea, may interact with anticoagulants and antiplatelet drugs: heparin, warfarin, aspirin, diclofenac, ibuprofen, enoxaparin. Antidiabetic medication. Herbs: angelica, clove, devil's claw, fenugreek, garlic, ginkgo, Panax ginseng, red clover, Siberian ginseng, turmeric.

GINKGO

Ginkgo biloba Herbal remedy, also known as Maidenhair.

Indications: Orally – for premenstrual syndrome, erectile dysfunction caused by serotonin reuptake inhibitors (SSRIs). Also primarily to improve memory, attention, cognitive function; as vasodilator to improve blood flow; for altitude sickness, Raynaud's syndrome.

Safety in pregnancy: Little recent evidence available, but generally considered unsafe to use in pregnancy. Leaf extract may cause miscarriage, antepartum haemorrhage, preterm labour. Colchinine content present in some combination products may contribute to birth defects – AVOID IN PRECONCEPTION PERIOD AND PREGNANCY. Use with caution at term – anticoagulant effect may prolong bleeding time. Caution: insufficient evidence of safety when breastfeeding.

Contraindications and precautions: Avoid when menstruating – plant oestrogens have an emmenagoguic effect that may cause menorrhagia. Avoid with haemorrhagic disorders, severe postpartum haemorrhage, retained products of conception; discontinue use for at least two weeks before elective surgery. Fruit pulp can cause severe allergic reactions. Avoid if allergic to poison ivy, mango rind, cashew shell oil. Do not consume crude ginkgo or seeds – can cause dyspnoea, convulsions, death.

Adverse effects: Skin irritation and rashes, nausea, vomiting, diarrhoea or constipation, dizziness and vertigo, headache, palpitations, bleeding disorders. May cause impaired fertility.

Interactions: Therapeutic oral doses, prolonged, excessive or inappropriate use may interact with anticoagulants and antiplatelet drugs: heparin, warfarin, aspirin, diclofenac, ibuprofen, enoxaparin. Also anticonvulsants, betablockers, some antihypertensives, diuretics, lipid-lowering agents, some antidepressants. Anticoagulant herbs: angelica, clove, garlic, ginger, ginkgo, meadowsweet, Panax ginseng, poplar, red clover, turmeric, willow bark.

GINSENG

Panax ginseng Herbal remedy, also known as Asian/Chinese/Korean red ginseng.

Indications: Orally – for stress, as immunostimulant, to improve cognitive function, aid memory, tone muscles; for depression, fatigue, anxiety, respiratory infections, various cancers. Also for erectile dysfunction, premature ejaculation. Used for various pregnancy disorders, menopausal symptoms.

Safety in pregnancy: AVOID IN PRECONCEPTION PERIOD AND PREGNANCY, especially the first trimester – ginsenoside Rb1 content may be teratogenic. Caution: insufficient information on safety when breastfeeding.

Contraindications and precautions: Avoid with diabetes mellitus, insomnia, coagulation or haemorrhagic disorders, oestrogen-dependent conditions – breast, cervical and ovarian cancer, endometriosis, fibroids. Do not confuse with Siberian ginseng.

Adverse effects: Insomnia, vaginal bleeding, mastalgia, hyper- or hypotension, oedema, diarrhoea, pruritus, headache, vertigo. Rare side effects include cholestatic hepatitis, anaphylactic shock, severe skin reactions.

Interactions: Therapeutic oral doses, prolonged, excessive or inappropriate use may interact with anticoagulants and antiplatelet drugs: heparin, warfarin, aspirin, diclofenac, ibuprofen, enoxaparin. Also oestrogens, antidiabetic medication, alcohol, caffeine, monoamine oxidase inhibitors, frusemide and other diuretics, immunosuppressants. Anticoagulant herbs: angelica, clove, garlic, ginger, ginkgo, meadowsweet, poplar, red clover, turmeric, willow bark. Hypoglycaemic herbs: bitter melon, fenugreek, ginger, kudzu, willow bark. Also Bitter orange, Ma huang.

GOLDENSEAL

Hydrastis canadensis Herbal remedy.

Indications: Orally – to aid labour and for postpartum haemorrhage. Also for the common cold, other respiratory infections, gastric ulcers, diarrhoea, constipation, mucous membrane inflammation, haemorrhoids. Topically for skin disorders; as an eye wash for conjunctivitis.

Safety in pregnancy: DO NOT USE IN PRECONCEPTION PERIOD, PREGNANCY OR BREASTFEEDING unless under the supervision of a qualified medical herbalist – contains berberine, thought to cross the placenta, may affect fetal development. Reports of kernicterus in neonates exposed to maternal goldenseal during breastfeeding. Do not use for babies, infants. Do not confuse with Echinacea which has many of the same properties; the two are often used together in non-pregnant people to enhance their immune-protective properties.

Contraindications and precautions: Avoid with any bleeding, diabetes mellitus, hypotension, hyper-bilirubinaemia. USA and Canada classify it as an endangered plant due to its popularity as a food supplement, which has led to overharvesting.

Adverse effects: Photosensitivity, diarrhoea or constipation, flatulence, vomiting, abdominal pain, distension; headache with large doses.

Interactions: Therapeutic oral doses, prolonged, excessive or inappropriate use may interact with anticoagulants and antiplatelet drugs: heparin, warfarin, aspirin, diclofenac, ibuprofen, enoxaparin. Also antidiabetic medication, antihypertensives, central nervous system depressants. Anticoagulant herbs: angelica, clove, garlic, ginger, ginkgo, meadowsweet, Panax ginseng, poplar, red clover, turmeric, willow bark. Hypoglycaemic herbs: bitter melon, devil's claw, fenugreek, garlic, horse chestnut, psyllium, Siberian ginseng. Hypotensive herbs: cat's claw, coenzyme Q10, fish oil, stinging nettle. Sedative herbs: calamus, California poppy, catnip, hops, Jamaican dogwood, kava, melatonin, sage, St John's wort, sassafras, skullcap.

GOTU KOLA
Centella asiatica (formerly *Hydrocotyle asiatica*) Herbal remedy.

Indications: Orally – for fatigue, anxiety, depression, memory and cognitive function; abdominal pain, diarrhoea, indigestion, peptic ulcer; varicose veins, thromboembolism, anaemia; colds, influenza, asthma; contraception, amenorrhoea, urinary tract infection. Topically – burns, wound healing, striae gravidarum, scars.

Safety in pregnancy: AVOID THERAPEUTIC ORAL DOSES IN PREGNANCY – risk of hepatotoxicity. Possibly safe used topically in small amounts under the supervision of a qualified medical herbalist.

Contraindications and precautions: Avoid with liver disease including obstetric cholestasis and with medication metabolized via the liver. Avoid with general anaesthetics, may cause depression of central nervous system when combined with systemic anaesthetics. Do not confuse with Cola nut/Kola nut.

Adverse effects: Gastric irritation, nausea, allergic contact dermatitis. Risk of hepatotoxicity with excessive or prolonged oral use (rare).

Interactions: Therapeutic oral doses, prolonged, excessive or inappropriate use may interact with sedatives, anaesthetics, carbamazepine, isoniazid, fluvastatin, niacin, tamoxifen, other hepatotoxic drugs. Hepatotoxic herbs: comfrey, pennyroyal oil, red yeast. Sedative herbs: California poppy, catnip, hops, Jamaican dogwood, kava, St John's wort, skullcap, valerian, yerba mansa.

GRAPEFRUIT
Citrus paradisi Herbal remedy.

Indications: Orally, fruit or juice – for asthma, weight loss, obesity, skin conditions, atherosclerosis. Seeds – as anti-infective agent. Topically or by inhalation – essential oil in aromatherapy used for pain relief, constipation, diarrhoea, nausea, vomiting; to uplift mood, as diuretic, anti-infective, anti-inflammatory, to reduce blood pressure.

Safety in pregnancy: Appears safe in amounts commonly used in foods. Essential oil used in aromatherapy is safe in doses up to 1.5% in pregnancy and 2% in labour and postnatal period.

Contraindications and precautions: Orally, topically or by inhalation – avoid if allergic to citrus fruit. Essential oil in aromatherapy – do not ingest. Avoid with threatened miscarriage, antepartum haemorrhage, excessive postpartum haemorrhage, retained products of conception – theoretical risk of anticoagulant effect. Do not use neat on skin or directly in a birthing pool. Use a diffuser for a maximum of 15–20 minutes in any hour; do not vaporize in the second stage of labour to avoid neonatal exposure; do not diffuse near neonates, elderly, ill people or those allergic to citrus fruit, including staff and visitors. Do not diffuse in public areas or use excessive amounts which spread to public areas of maternity unit, to avoid excessive exposure of the woman, baby, visitors and staff to potential adverse effects. Do not apply directly to breasts in postnatal period, or wash with water before the baby starts feeding to avoid adverse neonatal effects from ingestion. Discontinue use if any allergic reactions occur to avoid accumulative reaction to specific chemicals – may lead to anaphylactic shock in severe cases. Store essential oil in a refrigerator to avoid oxidation: shelf life of 3–6 months. Do not use in combination with homeopathic remedies or store with remedies. Excessive oral consumption of fruit or juice must be avoided with many drugs – check pharmacopoeia.

Adverse effects: Essential oil – skin sensitivity, photosensitivity, diarrhoea. Juice in large amounts – gastric irritation, diarrhoea, bruising, bleeding. Also ulcerative conditions with prolonged or excessive use, kidney stones, renal failure in extreme cases, possible increased risk of oestrogen-dependent cancers.

Interactions: Orally – general risk of impaired absorption and metabolism of many drugs. Therapeutic oral doses, including excessive consumption of fruit or juice, may interact with anticoagulants, antiplatelet drugs: heparin, warfarin, aspirin, diclofenac, ibuprofen, enoxaparin. Also antihypertensives, anticonvulsants, anticholesterol medication. Anticoagulant herbs: angelica, clove, garlic, ginger, ginkgo, meadowsweet, Panax ginseng, poplar, red clover, turmeric, willow bark.

GREEN TEA
Camellia sinensis Herbal remedy.

Indications: Orally – for cognitive performance, mental alertness, chronic fatigue syndrome, hypotension, headache, depression, nausea, vomiting, diarrhoea, ulcerative colitis, weight loss; human papilloma virus, genital and perianal warts, urinary tract infection, dental and mouth conditions, fractures, renal calculi; various cancers. Topically – for sunburn, as a compress for headache or tired eyes.

Safety in pregnancy: Considered safe in amounts commonly consumed in tea or used in therapeutic doses orally. Excessive consumption (more than 5–6 cups daily) increases miscarriage risk and folic acid deficiency-related birth defects, for example spina bifida, due to caffeine levels. Probably safe during breastfeeding – large amounts may cause neonatal irritability and diarrhoea.

Contraindications and precautions: Avoid with anaemia, may increase iron deficiency. May aggravate anxiety disorders due to caffeine content. Caffeine may affect platelets, prolonging bleeding times, avoid with threatened miscarriage, antepartum haemorrhage, systemic bruising. Reduce dose or eliminate if palpitations occur. Some research suggests caffeine in green tea affects insulin resistance, so avoid in diabetic women.

Adverse effects: Diarrhoea, nausea, skin rashes, insomnia, anaphylaxis. Excessive consumption may cause hypertension, hypotension, thrombocytopenic purpura, muscle pain, nervous irritability, hypokalaemia. Prolonged use may lead to irritable bowel syndrome, osteoporosis. Caffeinated green tea increases intraocular pressure. Hepatotoxicity rare, but serious. Abrupt discontinuation of green tea consumption may cause caffeine withdrawal symptoms, although controversial. Topical use of green tea – skin redness, inflammation, irritation, itching, burning. Excessive consumption may affect tests for bleeding time, urinary catecholamines, ferritin, glucose, iron, liver function tests, vanillyl mandelic acid tests for phaechromocytoma. May give false negative urinalysis reagent strip results when testing for sugar or occult blood.

Interactions: Therapeutic oral doses, including excessive consumption of tea as a nutritional aid, may interact with anticoagulant and antiplatelet drugs: heparin, warfarin, aspirin, diclofenac, ibuprofen, enoxaparin. Also alcohol, nicotine, amphetamines, ephedrine, cocaine, antidiabetic drugs, cimetidine, antipsychotic drugs, oestrogens, contraceptive Pill, monamine oxidase inhibitors, fluconazole, lithium, certain antihypertensives, quinolone antibiotics, theophylline, hepatotoxic drugs. Herbs: angelica, bitter orange, clove, garlic, ginger, ginkgo, ma huang (ephedra), Panax ginseng. Caffeine-containing plants: coffee, black tea, oolong tea, guarana, mate, cola. Also hepatotoxic herbs: bishop's weed, borage, uva ursi. Genistein-containing herbs in combination with caffeine may increase risk of abnormal cell growth: soy, kudzu, red clover, alfalfa. Also possibly calcium, folic acid, iron, magnesium.

HAMAMELIS, herbal remedy *see* **Witch hazel;**
see also **Hamamelis, homeopathic remedy**

HAMAMELIS

Hamamelis virginica Homeopathic remedy from witch hazel.

Obstetric indications: Topically – for haemorrhoids, varicosities in legs, vulva; phlebitis, epistaxis.

Key features: Congestion, swelling, bruised soreness; passive venous bleeding, weakness due to blood loss, feeling of fullness in nose, anus sore and raw, tired limbs, sore muscles, joints; prickling, stinging pain, very sensitive to touch.

Emotional symptoms: Feels lack of respect; irritability, depressed; feels isolated.

Better for: Fresh air; thinking; talking; reading.

Worse for: Warm, moist air; touch, pressure; movement; night-time.

Safety: Do not use in high potency in conjunction with homeopathic Arnica. Not generally used for wound healing – do not confuse with Hamamelis, herbal remedy. Do not use if there are any medical or obstetric complications. Not to be used as a replacement for standard medical care. Do not use with aromatherapy essential oils, topically or by inhalation, or with antacids, decongestants, laxatives or cough lozenges – inactivates the remedy. Do not take with food or drink. Do not take prophylactically – may lead to reverse proving. Should not be used by women who do not fit the symptom picture to avoid reverse proving. To be handled by the intended recipient only.

HAWTHORN
Crataegus monogyna, Crataegus laevigata Herbal remedy.

Indications: Orally – for hypotension, hypertension, to reduce cholesterol, as a sedative, antispasmodic, astringent, diuretic. Also for amenorrhoea, indigestion, diarrhoea, abdominal pain. Topically – for boils, sores, ulcers, itching skin.

Safety in pregnancy: Generally appears safe in non-pregnant individuals. Caution: insufficient information on safety in pregnancy and breastfeeding.

Contraindications and precautions: Avoid with any cardiovascular compromise including variations in blood pressure. Avoid prior to elective surgery.

Adverse effects: Abdominal pain, nausea, agitation, insomnia, dizziness, headache, fatigue, dyspnoea, skin irritation, tachycardia, palpitations.

Interactions: Major risk of interaction with vasodilatory drugs, including those for erectile dysfunction. Anticoagulants, antiplatelet drugs, antihypotensives. Anticoagulant herbs: angelica, clove, garlic, ginger, ginkgo, Panax ginseng. Hypotensive herbs: cat's claw, coenzyme Q10, fish oil, stinging nettle.

HEMP *see* Cannabis

HENBANE
Hyoscyamus niger Herbal remedy, also known as Black henbane, Stinking nightshade.

Indications: Orally – for constipation, oesophageal reflux, paralytic ileus. Topically – for scar tissue.

Safety in pregnancy: AVOID ORAL AND TOPICAL USE IN PREGNANCY – risk of toxicity.

Contraindications and precautions: Do not self-medicate, contains hyoscyamine and scopolamine, excessive doses can cause poisoning and death. Use only under the supervision of a qualified medical herbalist. Do not confuse with Belladonna, herbal remedy or Belladonna, homeopathic remedy, also from the nightshade family.

Adverse effects: Dry mouth, red skin, constipation, overheating with reduced sweating, visual disturbance, tachycardia, dysuria. Toxicity symptoms – restlessness, hallucinations, delirium, mania, then exhaustion, sleep, death by asphyxiation.

Interactions: Therapeutic oral doses, prolonged, excessive or inappropriate use may interact with anticholinergic drugs: antihistamines, atropine, belladonna, hyoscyamine, phenothiazines, procainamide, scopolamine, tricyclic antidepressants. Anticholinergic herbs: angel's trumpet, belladonna, deadly nightshade, European mandrake, scopolia.

HENNA
Lawsonia inermis Herbal remedy.

Indications: Orally – for gastrointestinal ulcers, headache. Topically – for dandruff, eczema, scabies, fungal infections, ulcers. Commonly used for henna "tattoos" including Hindu celebratory mehndi, and for hair colouring.

Safety in pregnancy: AVOID ORAL USE IN PREGNANCY – may cause miscarriage. Topical use for hair colouring appears safe in small amounts, possibly safer than standard hair colourings.

Contraindications and precautions: Avoid if henna sensitivity. Do not use on neonates – risk of anaemia in infants with hyper-bilirubinaemia and haemolysis in babies with glucose 6 phosphate dehydrogenase (G6PD) deficiency. If using for body tattoos or mehndi, ensure natural brown/red henna, not black henna which contains para-phenylenediamine – risk of severe skin irritation, blistering, burning.

Adverse effects: Orally – stomach upset. Topically – contact dermatitis, redness, itching, burning, swelling, blisters, excoriation, scarring. Excessive exposure, as with occupational use, may lead to urticaria, rhinitis, wheezing, bronchial asthma.

Interactions: Prolonged, excessive or inappropriate oral use may interact with lithium.

HIBISCUS
Hibiscus sabdariffa Herbal remedy, also known as Roselle, Rose of Sharon, China rose.

Indications: Orally – to promote lactation, stimulate menstruation, aid male fertility. Also for anxiety, poor appetite, respiratory and urinary tract infections, renal and bladder calculi, as a laxative and diuretic, for weight loss, anaemia, hypertension, hypercholesterolaemia, diabetes mellitus, cancer. Topically – for wound healing. Used in many traditional medicine cultures; used for contraception in Ayurvedic medicine.

Safety in pregnancy: AVOID IN PREGNANCY, including tea – may cause miscarriage. Use in labour and breastfeeding is safe enough in small amounts but (unproven) suggestion that excessive consumption reduces maternal fluid intake. Adverse effects on uterine muscle appear dose-dependent, either increasing or reducing contractility. Animal studies suggest excessive maternal consumption in pregnancy and breastfeeding may delay onset of puberty in female offspring, but no evidence yet of similar effects in humans.

Contraindications and precautions: Caution in labour – may cause hypertonic uterine action in large/prolonged doses; do not use in conjunction with oxytocic drugs or with essential oils and herbal remedies thought to trigger uterine contractions. Caution with commercially produced herbal teas containing several herbs, may contain hibiscus – check labels, including alternative names. Avoid in diabetes mellitus, may lower serum glucose. May reduce systolic blood pressure, caution with women with low blood pressure. May be toxic to animals, especially dogs.

Adverse effects: Orally – abdominal distension, flatulence, epigastric pain, nausea, dysuria, headache, tinnitus, hypoglycaemia, hypotension.

Interactions: Therapeutic oral doses, prolonged, excessive or inappropriate use may interact with paracetamol, oxytocics, antidiabetic drugs, antihypertensives, some antimalarials, amitriptyline, ondansetron, propranolol, theophylline, verapamil, dexamethasone, diazepam, diclofenac, ibuprofen, codeine, statins. Herbs: cat's claw, coenzyme Q10, chromium, devil's claw, fenugreek, fish oil, garlic, guar gum, L-arginine, lyceum, Panax ginseng, psyllium, Siberian ginseng, stinging nettle. Also possibly oral vitamin B12. Also oestrogenic herbs: black cohosh, blue cohosh, dong quai, evening primrose, fennel, fenugreek, ginkgo, ginseng, liquorice, raspberry leaf, red clover, vitex agnus castus.

HOLY BASIL

Ocimum tenuiflorum, Ocimum sanctum Herbal remedy.

Indications: Orally – for the common cold, influenza, diabetes mellitus, hypercholesterolaemia, hypertension, asthma, bronchitis, earache, headache, stomach upset, viral hepatitis, anxiety, stress, mercury poisoning, as mosquito repellent, antidote to snake and scorpion bites. Topically – ringworm, gingivitis, dental plaque. Used in traditional Chinese and Ayurvedic medicine.

Safety in pregnancy: Appears safe in amounts commonly used in foods. AVOID THERAPEUTIC ORAL USE IN PRECONCEPTION PERIOD AND

PREGNANCY – high doses may affect blastocyst implantation or cause miscarriage, preterm labour.

Contraindications and precautions: Coagulation and haemorrhagic disorders, thyroid disease, diabetes mellitus. Do not confuse with Basil.

Adverse effects: Nausea, vomiting, diarrhoea, inhibition of platelet aggregation with risk of bleeding, bruising.

Interactions: Therapeutic oral doses, prolonged, excessive or inappropriate use may interact with anticoagulants and antiplatelet drugs: heparin, warfarin, aspirin, diclofenac, ibuprofen, enoxaparin. Also antidiabetic medication, thyroid medication, barbiturates. Anticoagulant herbs: angelica, clove, garlic, ginger, ginkgo, Panax ginseng. Hypoglycaemic herbs: devil's claw, fenugreek, Siberian ginseng.

HOODIA

Hoodia gordonii Herbal remedy, also known as Cactus, Kalahari cactus.

Indications: Orally – appetite suppressant for obesity and weight loss.

Safety in pregnancy: Caution: insufficient information available, but conscious weight loss is not advised during pregnancy.

Contraindications and precautions: Avoid with hypertension, pre-existing or gestational diabetes, hepatic compromise, obstetric cholestasis. Do not confuse with prickly pear cactus.

Adverse effects: Nausea, vomiting, skin reactions, tachycardia, hypertension. May interfere with liver function.

Interactions: Therapeutic oral doses, prolonged, excessive or inappropriate use may interact with antidiabetic medication and hypoglycaemic herbs: devil's claw, fenugreek, Panax ginseng, Siberian ginseng.

HOPS

Humulus lupulus Herbal remedy.

Indications: Orally – to stimulate lactation, for menopausal symptoms, anxiety, insomnia, restlessness, nervousness, irritability, cystitis, indigestion, intestinal cramps; as an appetite stimulant, diuretic. Also for prostate, breast and ovarian cancer, hyperlipidaemia, neuralgia. Topically – for leg ulcers, postmenopausal vaginal atrophy, antibacterial.

Safety in pregnancy: Appears safe in amounts commonly used in foods. AVOID THERAPEUTIC DOSES IN PREGNANCY – contains plant oestrogens that may cause uterine contraction, leading to miscarriage, preterm labour.

Contraindications and precautions: Avoid with depression, oestrogen-dependent conditions – breast, ovarian and cervical cancer, endometriosis, fibroids. Caution – often combined with Valerian to aid sleep.

Adverse effects: Orally – dizziness, sedation, menstrual disturbances. Topically – allergic reactions, contact dermatitis. Inhalation – dry cough, dyspnoea, chronic bronchitis with prolonged use.

Interactions: Therapeutic oral doses, prolonged, excessive or inappropriate use may interact with alcohol, central nervous system depressants, theophylline, pentazocine, propranolol, imipramine, progesterones, oestrogens, caffeine, verapamil, glucocorticoids, fentanyl. Sedative herbs: calamus, California poppy, catnip, Jamaican dogwood, kava, St John's wort, skullcap, valerian, yerba mansa. Oestrogenic herbs: black cohosh, blue cohosh, dong quai, evening primrose, fennel, fenugreek, ginkgo, ginseng, liquorice, raspberry leaf, red clover, vitex agnus castus.

HORSE CHESTNUT
Aesculus hippocastanum Herbal remedy.

Indications: Orally – for varicose veins, haemorrhoids, phlebitis. Seeds used for diarrhoea, fever, chronic venous insufficiency, male infertility, irritable bowel syndrome. Bark – for malaria, dysentery. Leaf – for eczema, dysmenorrhoea, inflammation from fractures, concussion, cough, arthritis, joint pain. Topically – bark used for lupus and dermal ulcerative conditions.

Safety in pregnancy: AVOID RAW SEED, BARK, LEAF OR FLOWER IN PREGNANCY – esculin content may cause uterine contractions, leading to miscarriage, preterm labour. Recent evidence suggests commercial preparations made from seed, used under the supervision of a qualified medical herbalist, may be safe in small amounts in pregnancy – but advise women not to self-medicate.

Contraindications and precautions: Avoid with antepartum haemorrhage, bleeding haemorrhoids, generalized bruising, coagulation or haemorrhagic disorders, diabetes mellitus, inflammatory bowel conditions, hepatic conditions, latex allergy, renal disease. Discontinue two weeks prior to surgery.

Adverse effects: Orally – commercially produced therapeutic products using seed extract normally have toxic constituent esculin removed. Unprocessed products containing esculin – risk of significant toxicity including nausea, vomiting, diarrhoea, headache, dizziness, coma, weakness, pruritus, calf spasms, toxic neuropathy, paralysis, death.

Interactions: Therapeutic oral doses, prolonged, excessive or inappropriate use may interact with anticoagulants and antiplatelet drugs: heparin, warfarin, aspirin, diclofenac, ibuprofen, enoxaparin. Also antidiabetic medication, lithium. Anticoagulant herbs: angelica, clove, garlic, ginger, ginkgo, meadowsweet, Panax ginseng, red clover, turmeric. Hypoglycaemic herbs: chromium, devil's claw, fenugreek, psyllium, Siberian ginseng.

HUÁNG QI *see* **Astralgus**

HYPERICUM, herbal remedy *see* **St John's wort**

HYPERICUM

Hypericum perforatum Homeopathic remedy from St John's wort.

Obstetric indications: Primarily for injury, especially puncture wounds, surgery, dental extractions; burns. Afterpains from instrumental delivery. Sharp, shooting coccygeal pain post-delivery. Better indicated for deep wounds than homeopathic Calendula – allows deeper dermal layer to heal, prevents bacterial growth. Available as tincture combined with calendula (HyperCal™), useful for perineal trauma.

Key features: Sharp shooting pain from injury/wound out of proportion to degree of trauma; redness, swelling, throbbing, numbness; vertigo or sensation of being lifted upwards or falling.

Emotional symptoms: Shock; anxiety.

Better for: Lying quietly; tilting head backwards.

Worse for: Damp, cold conditions; warm, stuffy room; shooting pain recurs if touched.

Safety: Do not confuse with St John's wort, herbal remedy. Do not use if there are any medical or obstetric complications. Not to be used as a replacement for standard medical care. Do not use with aromatherapy essential oils, topically or by inhalation, or with antacids, decongestants, laxatives or cough lozenges – inactivates the remedy. Do not take with food or drink. Do not take prophylactically – may lead to reverse proving. Should not be used by women who do not fit the symptom picture to avoid reverse proving. To be handled by the intended recipient only.

HYSSOP

Hyssopus officinalis Herbal remedy.

Indications: Orally – for liver and gallbladder conditions, intestinal inflammation, coughs, common cold, sore throat, asthma, urinary tract infection, flatulence, colic, anorexia, poor circulation, HIV/AIDS, dysmenorrhoea, digestive and intestinal conditions. Topically – oil used in baths to induce sweating, on skin for dermatitis, burns, bruises, frostbite.

Safety in pregnancy: Appears safe in amounts commonly used in foods. AVOID THERAPEUTIC ORAL DOSES AND TOPICAL ESSENTIAL OIL IN PREGNANCY – may cause uterine stimulation, miscarriage, preterm labour. Caution: insufficient information on safety when breastfeeding.

Contraindications and precautions: Epilepsy, may increase fits. Do not ingest oil.

Adverse effects: Oral therapeutic doses and excessive essential oil use may cause toxicity leading to vomiting, quickly followed by epileptiform fits.

Interactions: Therapeutic oral doses, prolonged, excessive or inappropriate use may theoretically interact with anticoagulant herbs: angelica, clove, garlic, ginger, ginkgo, meadowsweet, Panax ginseng, poplar, red clover, turmeric.

INDIAN ELM *see* Slippery elm

INDIAN GINSENG *see* Ashwagandha

IPECACUANHA
Psychotria ipecacuanha, Cephaelis ipecacuanha Herbal remedy, also known as Brazil root.

Indications: Orally – as an emetic after overdose of toxic substances. Also as an expectorant, appetite stimulant, for croup, amoebic dysentery.

Safety in pregnancy: AVOID IN PREGNANCY – possible uterine stimulant, leading to miscarriage, preterm labour. Caution: no information on safety when breastfeeding.

Contraindications and precautions: Avoid with inflammatory gastrointestinal conditions, unconsciousness, poisoning with ingestion of corrosives, petroleum substances, strychnine.

Adverse effects: Excessive or prolonged use may lead to cardiomyopathies, anorexia; long-term abuse may trigger hypochondria and Munchausen syndrome.

Interactions: Activated charcoal, often given to absorb toxins from ingested poisons – also absorbs and inactivates ipecacuanha.

IPECACUANHA
Psychotria ipecacuanha Homeopathic remedy, known as ipecac.

Obstetric indications: Nausea, severe persistent or intermittently recurring, often unable to vomit; hyperemesis gravidarum with profuse vomiting, diarrhoea, headache. Labour pain, postpartum haemorrhage, headache with constant nausea.

Key features: Dislikes food, smell of food. Hot sweats or cold and clammy. Looks deathly, bluish, dark-ringed eyes.

Emotional symptoms: Changeable mood, anxious, angry, difficult to deal with.

Better for: Daytime.

Worse for: Night-time.

Safety: Do not use if there are any medical or obstetric complications. Not to be used as a replacement for standard medical care. Do not use with aromatherapy essential oils, topically or by inhalation, or with antacids, decongestants, laxatives or cough lozenges – inactivates the remedy. Do not take with food or drink. Do not take prophylactically – may lead to reverse proving. Should not be used by women who do not fit the symptom picture to avoid reverse proving. To be handled by the intended recipient only. Do not confuse with Ipecacuanha, herbal remedy.

ISIHLAMBEZO
Herbal remedy.

Indications: Orally – traditional Zulu remedy in South Africa, to prepare for birth, as abortifacient, to reduce oedema, to induce labour and aid progress, for intrapartum pain relief; to strengthen infant's bones. Thought to consist of up to 50 different plants, commonly including: natal lily/Kaffir lily (*Clivia miniate*), blue lily/African lily (*Agapanthus africanus*), wild verbena (*Pentanisia prunelloides*) and wild rhubarb (*Gunnera perpensa*), all of which are known uterotonics.

Safety in pregnancy: Safety is unknown but reports of serious adverse effects – advise women to avoid using. May cause miscarriage, preterm or precipitate labour, hypertonic uterine action.

Contraindications and precautions: Avoid with history of previous Caesarean section, other uterine scars, history of precipitate labour, antepartum haemorrhage. Avoid with uterotonic drugs or herbs to expedite labour. Avoid with obstructed labour, maternal medical or fetal abnormality conditions.

Adverse effects: Postpartum haemorrhage, uterine hypertonia or, conversely, cervical dystocia, fetal, neonatal or maternal death.

Interactions: Therapeutic oral doses, prolonged, excessive or inappropriate use may interact with anticoagulant herbs: angelica, clove, garlic, ginger, ginkgo, meadowsweet, Panax ginseng, poplar, red clover, turmeric. Oestrogenic herbs: black cohosh, blue cohosh, dong quai, evening primrose, fennel, fenugreek, ginkgo, ginseng, liquorice, raspberry leaf, red clover, vitex agnus castus.

ISPAGHULA
Plantago ovata Herbal remedy, also known as Blond psyllium.

Indications: Orally – for constipation, anal fissures, post-anorectal surgery, diarrhoea, irritable bowel syndrome, dysentery, colorectal cancer, Crohn's disease, ulcerative colitis, weight control. Topically – as a poultice for hair follicle abscess.

Safety in pregnancy: Appears safe, orally and topically, in therapeutic oral doses in pregnancy and breastfeeding.

Contraindications and precautions: Orally – advise women to drink plenty of water to avoid potential adverse effects, particularly dysphagia, oesophageal or colonic obstruction. Avoid in diabetes, gastrointestinal conditions, allergy to psyllium, hypotension.

Adverse effects: Flatulence, abdominal pain, diarrhoea, constipation, indigestion, nausea, bowel obstruction, allergic reactions, headache, backache, rhinitis, sinusitis.

Interactions: Therapeutic oral doses, prolonged, excessive or inappropriate use may interact with anticoagulants and antiplatelet drugs: heparin, warfarin, aspirin, diclofenac, ibuprofen, enoxaparin. Also antidiabetic medication, anticonvulsants, oestradiol, lithium. Hypoglycaemic herbs: bitter melon, chromium, devil's claw, fenugreek, garlic, horse chestnut, Panax ginseng, Siberian ginseng. Hypotensive herbs: cat's claw, coenzyme Q10, fish oil, stinging nettle. Iron, riboflavin – may affect absorption.

JASMINE
Jasminum officinale, Jasminum grandiflorum Herbal remedy, also known as Jati.

Indications: Orally – used in Ayurvedic medicine for abdominal pain, dysentery, as a sedative, hepatitis, cancer prevention. Also consumed as tea. Topically – essential oil in aromatherapy used for relaxation and stress relief, to initiate labour, for pain relief in labour, retained placenta, postnatal "blues", to suppress lactation (controversial), for skin diseases, wound healing, mouth ulcers, as an antispasmodic, aphrodisiac, antibacterial, antifungal, antiviral. By inhalation, essential oil – for stress, mental alertness, decreasing food cravings.

Safety in pregnancy: Appears safe in amounts commonly used in foods but advise cautious use of tea – contains caffeine, although amount depends on type of base tea used, highest with black tea, lowest with oolong tea. AVOID THERAPEUTIC ORAL DOSES IN PREGNANCY unless under the supervision of a qualified Ayurvedic practitioner. AVOID ESSENTIAL OIL TOPICALLY OR BY INHALATION IN PREGNANCY until term – emmenagoguic due to ketone content, potentially causing miscarriage, preterm labour.

Contraindications and precautions: Orally – tea contains caffeine, so apply same precautions as other caffeinated drinks – caution in pregnancy. Essential oil in aromatherapy – do not ingest. Avoid excessive use in well-established labour – uterine-contracting effect may cause hypertonic contractions. Do not use with oxytocic drugs or herbs to initiate or expedite labour including Black cohosh, Blue cohosh, Raspberry leaf, Red clover, Vitex agnus castus, Evening primrose oil. Do not use neat on skin or directly in a birthing pool. Caution in the postnatal period – emmenagoguic effect may precipitate postpartum haemorrhage, especially if retained products of conception. Do not apply directly to breasts in postnatal period, or wash with water before the baby starts feeding to avoid adverse neonatal effects from ingestion. Aroma can be overpowering to some. Use a diffuser for a maximum of 15–20 minutes in any hour; do not vaporize in the second stage of labour to avoid neonatal exposure; do not diffuse near neonates, elderly or ill people. Do not diffuse in public areas or use excessive amounts which spread to public areas of maternity unit, to avoid excessive exposure of the woman, baby, visitors and staff to potential adverse effects. Discontinue use if any allergic reactions occur to avoid accumulative reaction to specific chemicals – may lead to anaphylactic shock in severe cases. Do not use with or store near homeopathic remedies. Store essential oil in a refrigerator to avoid rapid oxidation. May be adulterated – purchase from a reputable company to ensure purity. Beware effect on women prone to hay fever or asthma triggered by flower pollen – may have psychosomatic effect. Not to be used by pregnant maternity staff caring for labouring women.

Adverse effects: Orally in therapeutic doses – none documented. Orally as tea – excessive consumption may cause caffeine-related headache, jitteriness, irritability, insomnia. Topically – skin irritation, hypersensitivity. By inhalation – headache, nausea.

Interactions: Essential oil, topically or by inhalation, prolonged, excessive or inappropriate use may interact with oxytocic drugs and oestrogenic herbs: black cohosh, blue cohosh, dong quai, evening primrose, fennel, fenugreek, ginkgo, ginseng, liquorice, raspberry leaf, red clover, vitex agnus castus. Other interactions related to type of tea used – see Green tea.

JATAMANSI *see* Spikenard

JATI *see* Jasmine

JEERA *see* Cumin

JUNIPER
Juniperus communis Herbal remedy.

Indications: Orally – for urinary tract infection, kidney and bladder stones, indigestion, flatulence, heartburn, abdominal bloating, loss of appetite, intestinal worms, diabetes mellitus, cancer. Topically – for rheumatic joint pain, inflammatory diseases, wounds. By inhalation – for pain relief, bronchitis.

Safety in pregnancy: AVOID ORAL USE AND ESSENTIAL OIL, TOPICALLY AND BY INHALATION, IN PREGNANCY, LABOUR AND POSTNATAL PERIOD – significant renal effects, may cause miscarriage due to poor implantation, preterm labour. Do not use near or for babies and children.

Contraindications and precautions: Avoid with renal disease, hyper- or hypotension, diabetes mellitus, coagulation and haemorrhagic conditions.

Adverse effects: Oral overdose can cause kidney pain and irritation, increased diuresis, proteinuria, haematuria, tachycardia, hypertension, convulsions, metrorrhagia, miscarriage. Topically – skin irritation and allergic reactions; with excessive use, renal damage.

Interactions: Therapeutic oral doses, prolonged, excessive or inappropriate use may interact with diuretics, antidiabetic medication. Antidiabetic herbs: devil's claw, fenugreek, guar gum, Panax ginseng, Siberian ginseng.

KALAHARI CACTUS *see* Hoodia

KALI CARBONICUM

Homeopathic remedy, tissue salt from potassium carbonate.

Obstetric indications: Failure to progress in labour with spasmodic, weak, ineffective contractions from back to pelvis into gluteal muscles; pain – cutting, darting, sharp, shooting, nagging. Occipito-posterior fetal position. Also for afterpains, backache, heartburn, indigestion, insomnia.

Key features: Weakness, headache in temple area, puffy eyelids. Very sensitive to cold, changes in weather. Recurrent respiratory problems: cough usually dry with wheezing or whooping. Heavy weight in pit of stomach, nausea, bloated sensation. Oedema of lower limbs. Dryness, burning sensations. Craves sweet foods, dislikes bread. Sensation of bed sinking into the floor.

Emotional symptoms: Very irritable, anxious, fear of future, failure, loss of control, being alone, death. Rigid thinking; strong sense of duty, behaving properly, obstinate. Easily startled, sensitive to noise.

Better for: Warmth; sitting up bent over; pressure applied to back; improves throughout day.

Worse for: Cold environment; hot drinks, coffee; lying down; exertion; touch; between 0200–0400 hours.

Safety: Do not confuse with potassium carbonate. Do not use if there are any medical or obstetric complications. Not to be used as a replacement for standard medical care. Do not use with aromatherapy essential oils, topically or by inhalation, or with antacids, decongestants, laxatives or cough lozenges – inactivates the remedy. Do not take with food or drink. Do not take prophylactically – may lead to reverse proving. Should not be used by women who do not fit the symptom picture to avoid reverse proving. To be handled by the intended recipient only.

KALI PHOS

Kalium phosphoricum Homeopathic remedy, tissue salt from potassium phosphate.

Obstetric indications: Backache in pregnancy. Failure to progress in labour with stitching, tearing, burning contractions often followed by depression, exhaustion.

Key features: Extreme physical and emotional exhaustion often due to overwork or anxiety. One-sided occipital headache. Empty, nervous feeling in abdomen. Profuse, thick yellow-orange discharges. Sensitive to cold with tendency to sweating.

Emotional symptoms: Anxiety, nervous dread, irritable, tearful, lethargic, depression, wishes to be alone. Brain weariness, loss of memory, shyness, reluctant to communicate with people. May be cruel to partner or baby.

Better for: Warmth; rest; nourishment; gentle movement; fresh air.

Worse for: Excitement; worry; mental and physical exertion; cold draughts.

Safety: Do not confuse with potassium phosphate. Do not use if there are any medical or obstetric complications. Not to be used as a replacement for standard medical care. Do not use with aromatherapy essential oils, topically or by inhalation, or with antacids, decongestants, laxatives or cough lozenges – inactivates the remedy. Do not take with food or drink. Do not take prophylactically – may lead to reverse proving. Should not be used by women who do not fit the symptom picture to avoid reverse proving. To be handled by the intended recipient only.

KAVA
Piper methysticum Herbal remedy.

Indications: Orally – for anxiety, stress, attention deficit-hyperactivity disorder, insomnia, benzodiazepine withdrawal, psychosis, depression, migraine, chronic fatigue syndrome, common cold, musculoskeletal pain, as an aphrodisiac. Also for urinary tract infection, uterine inflammation, sexually transmitted diseases, dysmenorrhoea, vaginal prolapse. Topically – for skin diseases, wound healing, as an analgesic, as a poultice for abscesses, mouthwash for toothache. Traditionally consumed as a social drink or smoked by some cultures for its euphoric effects. Banned in Europe and Canada.

Safety in pregnancy: AVOID IN PREGNANCY AND BREASTFEEDING – pyrone constituents may cause miscarriage, preterm labour, hypertonic uterine action, pass into breast milk.

Contraindications and precautions: Avoid with depression, liver compromise or hepatitis, Parkinson's disease. Caution with unanticipated abnormal liver function test results.

Adverse effects: Orally – gastrointestinal upset, headache, dizziness, drowsiness, enlarged pupils, dry mouth, allergic skin reactions, abnormal reflexes, twisting movements, acute urinary retention. Also hepatotoxicity, death, although disputed by some and may depend on how kava is prepared and from which part of the plant. Hepatotoxicity may be related to drinking kava tea with alcohol that further compromises liver function.

Interactions: Therapeutic oral doses, prolonged, excessive or inappropriate use may interact with central nervous system depressants: alcohol, barbiturates, benzodiazepines, etc.; tricyclic antidepressants, pentazocine, propranolol, theophylline, cimetidine, ranitidine, diazepam, phenytoin,   sterone, ibuprofen, diclofenac, corticosteroids. Also anticoagulants: heparin, warfarin, aspirin; antidiabetic medication, tamoxifen, ondansetron, tramadol, anaesthetics, erythromycin, chemotherapy drugs, drugs with risk of hepatotoxicity, alcohol. Hepatotoxic herbs: chaparral, comfrey, pennyroyal oil, red yeast. Sedative herbs: calamus, California poppy, catnip, hops, Jamaican dogwood, kava, St John's wort, skullcap, valerian, yerba mansa. Anticoagulant herbs: angelica, clove, fenugreek, feverfew, garlic, ginger, ginkgo, Panax ginseng, poplar, red clover, turmeric.

KELP

Fucus vesiculosus Algae from seaweed.

Indications: Orally – as food supplement, rich in antioxidants, vitamin C, manganese, zinc. Used medicinally to combat oxidative stress, aid cardiovascular health. Commonly found in commercial products, often containing multiple ingredients.

Safety in pregnancy: AVOID ORAL USE IN PREGNANCY – high levels of iodine. AVOID TOPICAL USE – risk of infection, especially when administered intravaginally.

Contraindications and precautions: Thyroid disease. See also Laminaria.

Adverse effects: Orally – gastrointestinal and renal disorders.

Interactions: Therapeutic oral doses, prolonged, excessive or inappropriate use may theoretically interact with anticoagulants: heparin, warfarin, aspirin, enoxaparin. Also antithyroid medication, lithium, various other drugs. Anticoagulant herbs: angelica, clove, fenugreek, feverfew, garlic, ginger, ginkgo, Panax ginseng, poplar, red clover, turmeric.

KHAT

Catha edulis, Celastrus edulis Herbal remedy.

Indications: Orally – to facilitate labour, for male fertility issues, diabetes mellitus, muscle strength, depression, fatigue, obesity, gastric ulcers, headache. Also chewed for recreational purposes, and to decrease libido, increase euphoria and aggression. Illegal in the UK and USA.

Safety in pregnancy: AVOID IN PREGNANCY AND BREASTFEEDING – may reduce maternal appetite, cause psychological dependence, reduce lactation.

Contraindications and precautions: Hypertension, depression, diabetes mellitus.

Adverse effects: In pregnancy, may cause poor maternal weight gain, poor placental perfusion, intrauterine growth retardation; maternal tachycardia, chest pain, hypertension. Appears to reduce lactation; some constituents metabolize to psycho-stimulating chemicals similar to ephedrine. Also euphoria, hyperactivity, aggression, anxiety, hypertension, tachycardia, mania, depression, paranoia, psyc... migraine, cerebral haemorrhage, myocardial infarction, pulmonary oedema, hepatic cirrhosis, encephalopathy.

Interactions: Serious risk of interaction with amoxycillin. Also therapeutic doses, if chewed and swallowed, as well as prolonged, excessive or inappropriate use, may interact with antihypertensives, antimalarials, monoamine oxidase inhibitors, stimulant drugs: cocaine, nicotine, amphetamines. Herbs: caffeine, cola nut, ephedra, guarana, yerba mate.

KLIP DAGGA *see* **Motherwort**

KOLA NUT *see* **Cola nut**

KOMBU *see* **Laminaria**

KOREAN RED GINSENG *see* **Ginseng**

KUDZU
Pueraria montana, Pueraria lobata Herbal remedy, also known as Ge gen.

Indications: Orally – to stimulate abortion, aid lactation, for menopausal symptoms. Commonly for alcohol hangover symptoms – headache, upset stomach, dizziness, vomiting and for alcoholism. Also for menopausal symptoms, weight loss, measles, dysentery, diarrhoea, allergic rhinitis, influenza, neck stiffness, migraine, deafness, diabetes mellitus, traumatic injuries, urticaria, pruritus, psoriasis.

Safety in pregnancy: AVOID IN PRECONCEPTION PERIOD AND EARLY PREGNANCY – human research suggests up to a 50% miscarriage rate. Caution: insufficient information on safety when breastfeeding; advise consultation with a qualified Chinese medicine practitioner.

Contraindications and precautions: Diabetes mellitus, coagulation and haemorrhagic disorders, hormone-sensitive conditions – ovarian, uterine and breast cancer, endometriosis, fibroids. Hepatic conditions.

Adverse effects: Urticaria, dizziness, nausea, indigestion, abdominal bloating, palpitations, allergic reaction, hangover-like symptoms, especially if taken prior to or with alcohol.

Interactions: Therapeutic oral doses, prolonged, excessive or inappropriate use may interact with contraceptive Pill, oestrogens, tamoxifen, anticoagulants, antiplatelet drugs: heparin, warfarin, aspirin, enoxaparin. Also antidiabetic medication, hepatotoxic drugs. Anticoagulant herbs: angelica, clove, fenugreek, feverfew, garlic, ginger, ginkgo, Panax ginseng, poplar, turmeric. Hepatotoxic herbs: chaparral, comfrey, pennyroyal oil, red yeast. Hypoglycaemic herbs: bitter melon, cassia cinnamon, chromium, devil's claw, horse chestnut, psyllium,

Siberian ginseng. Oestrogenic herbs: black cohosh, blue cohosh, dong quai, evening primrose, fennel, liquorice, raspberry leaf, red clover, vitex agnus castus.

LADY'S MANTLE

Alchemilla vulgaris Herbal remedy, also known as Alchemilla.

Indications: Orally – for dysmenorrhoea, menorrhagia; abnormal vaginal discharge, infections and prolapse; uterine fibroids, endometriosis, infertility, menopausal hot flushes, postnatal uterine wound healing. Also as a diuretic, antispasmodic, for skin conditions, insomnia, diarrhoea, haemorrhoids. Gel from leaves used for mouth ulcers.

Safety in pregnancy: Caution: no information available on safety. Advise women not to self-medicate, consult a qualified medical herbalist.

Contraindications and precautions: Astringent properties may theoretically increase blood pressure.

Adverse effects: Tannin content may impair iron and zinc absorption, cause constipation and, in large amounts, potentially decrease clotting times. May be hepatotoxic in large amounts.

Interactions: Therapeutic oral doses, prolonged, excessive or inappropriate use may interact with absorption of oral medicines due to high tannin levels.

LADY'S SLIPPER *see* Nerve root

LAMINARIA

Laminaria digitata, *Laminaria japonica* Algae from seaweed, also known as Kombu.

Indications: Topically – as intracervical "tent" to aid cervical ripening in pregnancy, to facilitate labour, induce abortion. Previously used medically to aid cervical dilation prior to curettage, removal of intrauterine devices, intravaginal diagnostic procedures, to facilitate intrauterine placement of therapeutic radium. Orally – for weight loss, as a laxative, to prevent cancer, for hypertension, radioactive intoxication.

Safety in pregnancy: Appears safe in amounts commonly used in foods. AVOID INTRACERVICAL USE IN PREGNANCY – increased risk of vaginal infection, bleeding. AVOID IN BREASTFEEDING – risk of toxicity. AVOID THERAPEUTIC ORAL DOSES IN PREGNANCY AND BREASTFEEDING – significant iron and arsenic levels may be toxic.

Contraindications and precautions: Thyroid conditions, serum iron disorders. See also Kelp.

Adverse effects: Intracervical "tents" associated with fetal distress, hypoxia, intrapartum stillbirth, neonatal sepsis, maternal pelvic cramps, cervical bleeding, rupture of cervical wall, hypertonic uterine action, later endometriosis. Orally – acne, exacerbation of thyroid disorders, allergic reactions.

Interactions: Therapeutic oral doses, prolonged, excessive or inappropriate use may interact with diuretics, iron supplements, ACE inhibitors, digoxin.

LARKSPUR *see* Staphysagria

LAVENDER
Lavendula angustifolia, Lavandula officinalis Herbal remedy.

Indications: Orally – for anxiety, depression, anorexia, flatulence, heartburn, nausea, vomiting, pain relief, antibacterial, acne, amenorrhoea. Topically – essential oil used in aromatherapy for pain relief, constipation, relaxation and stress relief, insomnia, skin conditions, to reduce inflammation, reduce blood pressure, relax muscles, as an antibacterial agent, for burns, scalds. Topically in water – for perineal wound healing, pain relief, prevention of infection. By inhalation – essential oil used for insomnia, anxiety, stress, fatigue, to aid labour onset, relieve intrapartum pain, postoperative nausea, headache, backache, sciatica, carpal tunnel syndrome, mild to moderate hypertension, colds and influenza, sinus congestion, constipation. Also for dysmenorrhoea, menopausal symptoms.

Safety in pregnancy: Essential oil in aromatherapy generally considered safe in pregnancy, labour, breastfeeding. Use sparingly in first trimester – may have slight oestrogenic effect; maximum dose 1.5% in second and third trimester; appears safe in doses up to 2% in labour and postnatally. Orally – appears safe in small amounts used in foods or in therapeutic doses under the supervision of a qualified medical herbalist.

Contraindications and precautions: Do not take internally unless under the supervision of a qualified medical herbalist. Essential oil, topically or by inhalation – avoid with low blood pressure; caution in the second trimester with physiological hypotension/postural hypotension; avoid in labour with epidural anaesthesia. Avoid with severe hypertension or fulminating pre-eclampsia, especially if on antihypertensive medication. Do not use neat on skin or open wounds, such as the perineum; do not use intravaginally. Do not use essential oil directly in a birthing pool. Discontinue use if skin reactions occur. Avoid in women prone to hay fever and asthma caused by flowers – although no pollen is present in essential oil, it may have a psychosomatic effect. Use a diffuser for a maximum of 15–20 minutes in any hour; do not diffuse in the second stage of labour to avoid neonatal exposure; do not diffuse near elderly or ill people. Do not diffuse near cats – toxic. Do not diffuse in public areas or use excessive amounts which spread to public areas of maternity unit, to avoid excessive exposure of the woman, baby, visitors and staff to potential adverse effects. Discontinue use if any allergic reactions occur to avoid accumulative reaction to specific chemicals – may lead to anaphylactic shock in severe cases. Do not use with or store near homeopathic remedies. Store in a refrigerator to avoid rapid oxidation. Do not confuse with spike lavender (*Lavandula stoechas*) or other types of lavender that may contain higher levels of chemicals that are potentially hazardous in pregnancy. Do not confuse with lavender cotton (*Santolina chamaecyparissus*).

Adverse effects: Topically – allergic contact dermatitis. Excessive use in labour may cause sedative effects in the mother, staff and visitors. By inhalation – allergic reactions, hay fever or asthmatic attacks in susceptible people. Orally – diarrhoea, constipation, headache, increased appetite. May have mild oestrogenic effects – gynaecomastia reported in pre-pubertal boys exposed to high doses of lavender oil or essence (as in environmental diffusion).

Interactions: Excessive use of essential oil, topically or by inhalation, may interact with antihypertensives and other drugs with hypotensive effect, for example bupivacaine; may theoretically also interact with sedatives, other drugs, herbs or essential oils with sedative effects. Therapeutic oral doses, prolonged, excessive or inappropriate use may interact with antihypertensives, antihistamines, tricyclic antidepressants, barbiturates, benzodiazepines. Antihypotensive herbs: cat's claw, coenzyme Q10, fish oil, stinging nettle. Sedative herbs: calamus, California poppy, catnip, hops, Jamaican dogwood, kava, St John's wort, skullcap, valerian, yerba mansa.

LEMON BALM
Melissa officinalis Herbal remedy, also known as Melissa.

Indications: Orally – in therapeutic doses, or as tea, for anxiety, stress, insomnia, depression, irritability, attention deficit-hyperactivity disorder, cognitive function, nausea and vomiting, heartburn, flatulence, irritable bowel syndrome, colic, headache, toothache, dysmenorrhoea, insect bites, chronic bronchitis, hypertension. Topically and by inhalation in aromatherapy – for cold sores, dementia.

Safety in pregnancy: Appears safe in amounts commonly used in foods and in small amounts as a tea. Essential oil used in aromatherapy appears safe in doses up to 1.5% in pregnancy and 2% in labour and postnatal period.

Contraindications and precautions: Orally – diabetes mellitus, anaesthesia, thyroid disease. Do not take therapeutic doses internally unless under the supervision of a qualified medical herbalist. Essential oil – do not use neat on skin or open wounds. Discontinue use if skin reactions occur. Store essential oil in a refrigerator to avoid rapid oxidation. Not to be used for neonates; do not vaporize in a baby's room; advise not to be diffused for longer than 15–20 minutes; do not diffuse near elderly or ill people. Do not use in combination with homeopathic remedies or store with remedies. May interfere with thyroid function test results. Do not confuse with Lemongrass. Do not confuse with other members of the mint family such as Peppermint, Pennyroyal.

Adverse effects: Orally – increased appetite, nausea, vomiting, abdominal pain, dizziness, wheezing, dysuria, hypoglycaemia. Topically – skin irritation, exacerbation of herpes symptoms.

Interactions: Therapeutic oral doses, prolonged, excessive or inappropriate use may interact with antidiabetic medication, alcohol, anaesthetics, central nervous system depressants, thyroid medication. Hypoglycaemic herbs: bitter melon, chromium, devil's claw, fenugreek, garlic, guar gum, horse chestnut, Panax ginseng, psyllium, Siberian ginseng. Sedative herbs: calamus, California poppy, catnip, hops, Jamaican dogwood, kava, St John's wort, skullcap, valerian, yerba mansa. Thyroid-suppressing herbs: bugleweed, wild thyme.

LEMONGRASS

Cymbopogon citratus, *Andropogon citratus* Herbal remedy.

Indications: Orally – for abdominal discomfort, nausea, vomiting, hypertension, musculoskeletal pain, neuralgia, common cold, cough, fatigue, as a sedative, antiseptic, mild astringent. Also as tea for health and wellbeing, infection prevention. Topically – essential oil used in aromatherapy for labour pain, headache, abdominal pain, musculoskeletal pain, antibacterial. By inhalation in aromatherapy for musculoskeletal pain, influenza, common cold. Popular in Ayurvedic medicine.

Safety in pregnancy: Appears safe in amounts commonly used in foods. AVOID EXCESSIVE CONSUMPTION OF TEA AND THERAPEUTIC ORAL DOSES IN PREGNANCY unless under the supervision of a qualified practitioner. AVOID ESSENTIAL OIL TOPICALLY OR BY INHALATION IN PREGNANCY – may have emmenagoguic, uterine-contracting properties, leading to threatened miscarriage, antepartum haemorrhage, preterm labour. Essential oil appears safe topically and by inhalation in labour and postnatal period in doses up to 2%.

Contraindications and precautions: Orally, topically or by inhalation – do not use in labour or postnatally if there is a known allergy to lemongrass. May interfere with bilirubin test results (maternal). Essential oil – do not use neat on skin; do not use in a birthing pool. Avoid with pre-existing or gestational diabetes, hepatic disease, antenatal obstetric cholestasis. Inhalation via a diffuser should be for no more than 15–20 minutes in any hour; do not vaporize near neonates, elderly or ill people. Do not use orally, topically or by inhalation if the mother receives pethidine or morphine. Menstruating maternity staff and visitors with labouring women using essential oil may experience menorrhagia; pregnant staff should avoid essential oil when caring for labouring women. Store essential oil in a refrigerator to avoid rapid oxidization. Do not use or store with homeopathic remedies. Do not confuse with Lemon balm.

Adverse effects: Skin irritation and rash from excessive oral or topical use. Allergic reactions, including dyspnoea, chest pain, throat swelling. May lower blood sugar levels.

Interactions: Therapeutic oral doses, prolonged, excessive or inappropriate use may interact with morphine, pethidine, theophylline, amitriptyline, citalopram, ondansetron, prednisolone, sertraline.

LEOPARD'S BANE *see* Arnica, herbal remedy, homeopathic remedy

LEVANT BERRY *see* Cocculus

LIME
Citrus aurantifolia Herbal remedy.

Indications: Topically – essential oil in aromatherapy, as a stimulant, antiseptic, for nausea, constipation, diarrhoea, heartburn, irritable bowel syndrome; to increase mental awareness, enhance mood, as an anti-inflammatory, antispasmodic, antipyrexial; for relaxation, stress, anxiety, to reduce mild hypertension. Orally – as food supplement, therapeutically for dysentery.

Safety in pregnancy: Essential oil appears safe in pregnancy, orally and topically in doses up to 1% in pregnancy and 2% in labour and postnatal period. Oral use safe in amounts commonly found in foods and in therapeutic doses.

Contraindications and precautions: Orally, topically, by inhalation – avoid with known citrus fruit allergy. Topically, essential oil – avoid exposure of skin to direct sunlight for at least 2 hours after topical administration; caution with hypertensive women. Do not ingest. Do not use neat on skin or directly in a birthing pool. Use a diffuser for a maximum of 15–20 minutes in any hour; do not vaporize in the second stage of labour to avoid neonatal exposure; do not diffuse near neonates, elderly, ill people or those allergic to citrus fruit. Do not diffuse near animals – toxic to cats and dogs. Do not diffuse in public areas or use excessive amounts which spread to public areas of maternity unit, to avoid excessive exposure of the woman, baby, visitors and staff to potential adverse effects. Discontinue use if any allergic reactions occur to avoid accumulative reaction to specific chemicals – may lead to anaphylactic shock in severe cases. Do not use with or store near homeopathic remedies. Store in a refrigerator to avoid rapid oxidation – shelf life of 3–6 months.

Adverse effects: Topically – photosensitivity, skin irritation, other allergic reactions. Orally – diarrhoea.

Interactions: Therapeutic oral doses, prolonged, excessive or inappropriate topical use may theoretically interact with photosensitizing drugs, for example chlorpromazine, and herbs: angelica, anise, bergamot oil, celery seed, St John's wort.

LINSEED *see* Flaxseed

LION'S TAIL, LION'S EAR *see* **Motherwort**

LIQUORICE
Glycyrrhiza glabra Herbal remedy.

Indications: Orally – for gastrointestinal ulcers, heartburn, colic, dry mouth, sore throat, cough, bronchitis, menopausal symptoms, bacterial and viral infections, cholestatic liver disorders, abscesses, food poisoning, chronic fatigue syndrome, postoperative recovery, contact dermatitis, hypercholesterolaemia, skin conditions. Available in commercially prepared products in combination with Siberian ginseng and Schisandra, Slippery elm or peony to treat various disorders. Topically – as a shampoo to reduce sebum secretion, as a gel for eczema, and to stem bleeding, as a topical cream for psoriasis, weight loss, as a gargle for postoperative recovery, as a paste for dental plaque. Also root chewed as a nutritional supplement.

Safety in pregnancy: AVOID THERAPEUTIC ORAL DOSES IN PRECONCEPTION PERIOD, PREGNANCY, LABOUR AND POSTNATAL PERIOD – abortifacient, oestrogenic, may cause miscarriage, preterm labour, hypertonic uterine action in term labour, fetal distress. High salt content may cause or exacerbate existing hypertension. Babies of women who consume excessive amounts in pregnancy may have raised cortisol levels due to glycyrrhizin content.

Contraindications and precautions: Avoid with gestational or essential hypertension, pre-eclampsia, high dietary salt intake, renal conditions, disturbed electrolytes, hormone-sensitive conditions – breast, uterine and cervical cancer, endometriosis, fibroids. Discontinue at least two weeks before elective surgery. Do not use for babies or children.

Adverse effects: Orally – nausea, vomiting, headaches, oedema, decreased libido in men. Excessive or prolonged use – hypertension, hypokalaemia due to high sodium content. In extreme cases, thrombocytopaenia, alkalosis, paralysis, ventricular tachycardia, encephalopathy, renal failure, cardiac arrest, even in previously healthy people. Chewing fibrous root without thorough mastication can lead to bowel obstruction. Topically – contact dermatitis. May affect test results for blood pressure and potassium.

Interactions: Therapeutic oral doses, prolonged, excessive or inappropriate use may interact with antihypertensives, corticosteroids, barbiturates, dexamethasone, diazepam, non-steroidal anti-inflammatories, for example diclofenac, ibuprofen; certain antidiabetic medication, phenytoin, anticoagulants: heparin, warfarin, aspirin, enoxaparin. Also cyclosporine, digoxin, diuretics, oestrogens. Stimulant laxative herbs: alder buckthorn, aloe vera, black root, blue flag, butternut bark, European buckthorn, greater bindweed, rhubarb, senna, yellow dock. Also digitalis, lily of the valley, pheasant's eye, squill, grapefruit juice, salt. Anticoagulant herbs: angelica, garlic, ginger, ginkgo, Panax ginseng, red clover, turmeric, willow.

LUCERNE *see* Alfalfa

LYCOPODIUM

Lycopodium clavatum Homeopathic remedy, also known as Club moss or Wolf's claw.

Obstetric indications: Flatulence, constipation. Insomnia. Failure to progress in labour: weak, erratic contractions, tearing, pressing, stinging, moving up from right to left. Weeps whilst walking around; obtains relief by pressing and relaxing foot alternately against firm surface, for example end of bed.

Key features: Mental, physical weakness; symptoms move from right to left. Tight, bloated abdomen; excessive flatulence but emptiness in stomach, constipation. Ravenous, not relieved by eating; desires sweet foods. Brick red, sandy sediment in urine; current or history of renal calculi; dryness of mucous membranes; pulsating sensation.

Emotional symptoms: Fear of failure, the future; hates to be contradicted, but full of contradictions; inferiority complex, but dictatorial, malicious, confused, irritable. Fears being alone but hates crowds; having someone in the next room is preferable.

Better for: Warm drinks, food; belching; passing urine; after midnight; open air; lying on left side; gentle exercise; loose clothing.

Worse for: Between 1600–2000 hours; pressure of clothes; overeating, milk, onions; windy weather; heat; warm room; right side.

Safety: Do not use if there are any medical or obstetric complications. Not to be used as a replacement for standard medical care. Do not use with aromatherapy essential oils, topically or by inhalation, or with antacids, decongestants, laxatives or cough lozenges – inactivates the remedy. Do not take with food or drink. Do not take prophylactically – may lead to reverse proving. Should not be used by women who do not fit the symptom picture to avoid reverse proving. To be handled by the intended recipient only. Do not confuse with Club moss, herbal remedy.

MA HUANG

Ephedra sinica, Ephedra vulgaris Herbal remedy, also known as Ephedra, Yellow horse.

Indications: Orally – for nasal congestion, asthma, bronchitis, colds, influenza, headache. Also for weight loss, allergies, nephritis, joint and bone pain, to enhance athletic performance. Traditionally used in Chinese medicine for 2000 years.

Safety in pregnancy: AVOID IN PRECONCEPTION PERIOD, PREGNANCY, LABOUR AND BREASTFEEDING – ephedrine and pseudoephedrine constituents are mutagenic, hepatotoxic, pose serious risk of severe adverse effects.

Contraindications and precautions: All ephedra-containing products are banned or statutorily regulated as controlled drugs in many countries. Avoid all use, especially with diabetes mellitus, hypertension, cardiac disease, anxiety syndromes, epilepsy, renal calculi, hepatic disease, thyroid disease. Do not confuse with alkaloid-free Mormon tea (*Ephedra nevadensis*).

Adverse effects: Orally – severe life-threatening effects including dizziness, restlessness, anxiety, irritability, personality changes, difficulty concentrating, insomnia, headache, increased thirst, dry mouth, nausea, vomiting, heartburn, tingling. Prolonged or excessive use can cause tachycardia, palpitations, hyperthermia, hypertension, myocardial infarction, subarachnoid haemorrhage, fits, psychosis. Long-term use can lead to dependence.

Interactions: Any significant oral use may interact with caffeine, theophylline, anticonvulsants, antidiabetic drugs, adrenaline, amphetamines, monoamine oxidase inhibitors, naproxen, ondansetron, propranolol, verapamil, dexamethasone, ergot derivatives, drugs with risk of hepatotoxicity. Herbs containing caffeine: black tea, coffee, cola nut, ergot, green tea, guarana, yerba mate. Hepatotoxic herbs: chaparral, comfrey, pennyroyal oil, red yeast. Also Panax ginseng. May interfere with thyroid function tests.

MABELE *see* **Calabash chalk**

MACE *see* **Nutmeg**

MAIDENHAIR *see* **Ginkgo**

MANDARIN
Citrus reticulata, Citrus nobilis Herbal remedy.

Indications: Topically – essential oil, also known as tangerine, used in aromatherapy for relaxation, to lift mood, ease fear, for anxiety, constipation, diarrhoea, irritable bowel syndrome, to reduce oedema, aid weight loss, treat skin conditions, prevent striae gravidarum, as an antibacterial, antifungal agent, diuretic, antispasmodic. Orally – peel used for asthma, heartburn, irritable bowel syndrome, cancer prevention, as a nutritional supplement.

Safety in pregnancy: Topically, essential oil in aromatherapy safe in doses up to 1.5% in pregnancy and 2% in labour and postnatal period. Orally – appears safe in amounts commonly used in foods.

Contraindications and precautions: Orally, topically and by inhalation – avoid if known allergy to citrus fruit. Essential oil, topically or by inhalation – mild anticoagulant effect; avoid with threatened miscarriage, antepartum haemorrhage, excessive postnatal lochia, with anticoagulants or preventative drugs with anticoagulant effect. Avoid exposure of skin to direct sunlight for at least 2 hours after topical administration. Do not ingest. Do not use neat on skin or directly in a birthing pool. Use a diffuser for a maximum of 15–20 minutes in any hour; do not vaporize in the second stage of labour to avoid neonatal exposure; do not diffuse near neonates, elderly, ill people or those allergic to citrus fruit. Do not diffuse near animals – toxic to cats and dogs. Do not diffuse in public areas or use excessive amounts which spread to public areas of maternity unit, to avoid excessive exposure of the woman, baby, visitors and staff to potential adverse effects. Discontinue use if any allergic reactions occur to avoid accumulative reaction to specific chemicals – may lead to anaphylactic shock in severe cases. Store in a refrigerator to avoid rapid oxidization; shelf life of 3–6 months; discard old or oxidized oils. Do not use in combination with homeopathic remedies or store with remedies.

Adverse effects: Skin irritation, photosensitivity.

Interactions: Theoretically, therapeutic oral doses, including excessive consumption of fruit juice, may interact with anticoagulants, ondansetron, citalopram, sertraline.

MARIGOLD

Tagetes erecta Herbal remedy, also known as African marigold, tagete.

Indications: Orally – to stimulate menstrual flow, prevent miscarriage, for mastitis, colic, flatulence, to aid bile flow, as an appetite stimulant, diuretic. Also for coughs, colds, mumps, sore eyes, dysentery, to induce sweating. Topically – for sores, ulcers, eczema, as a mosquito repellent.

Safety in pregnancy: Appears safe in amounts commonly found in foods. Advise caution: little information available on safety of therapeutic doses in pregnancy and breastfeeding.

Contraindications and precautions: Avoid if sensitive to plants in the Asteraceae/Compositae family – ragweed, chrysanthemums, marigolds, daisies. Do not confuse with Calendula or Marsh marigold.

Adverse effects: Topically – contact dermatitis, allergic reactions.

Interactions: None documented.

MARIJUANA *see* Cannabis

MARJORAM

Origanum majorana, Majorana majorana Herbal remedy, also known as Sweet marjoram.

Indications: Orally – for rhinitis, cough, common cold, other viral and bacterial infections, gastric ulcers, flatulence, liver disease, gallstones, depression, mood swings, dysmenorrhoea, menopausal symptoms, dizziness, headaches, migraines, paralysis, epilepsy, hypertension, diabetes mellitus, cardiac arrhythmias, to stimulate appetite, promote lactation, improve circulation. Topically and by inhalation – essential oil in aromatherapy used for painful joints, sore muscles, sprains, bruises, backache, insomnia, stress, mood swings, headache, to promote lactation.

Safety in pregnancy: Appears safe in amounts commonly used in foods. AVOID THERAPEUTIC ORAL DOSES AND TOPICAL USE OF ESSENTIAL OIL IN PREGNANCY – emmenagoguic, potentially increasing risk of miscarriage, antepartum haemorrhage, preterm labour. Essential oil appears safe for use in term labour and breastfeeding in doses up to 2%.

Contraindications and precautions: Orally, topically and by inhalation – avoid if allergic to plants in the Lamiaceae family – basil, hyssop, lavender, mint, oregano, sage, clary sage. Discontinue oral therapeutic doses prior to surgery – increased risk of bleeding. Avoid essential oil and oral therapeutic doses with epilepsy, fulminating pre-eclampsia – possible increased risk of fits. Essential oil, intrapartum and postnatally in aromatherapy – do not ingest essential oil; do not apply neat; do not use topically on breasts to stimulate lactation; do not add direct to a birthing pool. Not for use on or near neonates; do not diffuse in public areas of a maternity unit, in a baby's room or near elderly or ill people. Store in a refrigerator; do not store with or use with homeopathic remedies. Do not confuse with Oregano.

Adverse effects: Topical and oral – skin irritation, skin lightening. May be toxic if taken orally in excess amounts – potentially carcinogenic, hepatotoxic.

Interactions: Therapeutic oral doses and, theoretically, prolonged, excessive or inappropriate use of essential oil may interact with anticoagulants and antiplatelet drugs: heparin, warfarin, aspirin, enoxaparin. Also atropine and other anticholinergic drugs. Anticoagulant herbs: angelica, garlic, ginger, ginkgo, Panax ginseng, red clover, turmeric, willow.

MARSHMALLOW

Althaea officinalis Herbal remedy.

Indications: Orally – for inflammation of respiratory and gastric mucous membranes, dry cough, diarrhoea, peptic ulcers, constipation, urinary tract inflammation, renal calculi. Topically – for abscesses, varicose and thrombotic ulcers, breast engorgement during breastfeeding, skin inflammation, burns, insect bites.

Safety in pregnancy: Very little information available, but given its potential to interact with anticoagulants, the advice is to AVOID THERAPEUTIC ORAL DOSES IN PRECONCEPTION PERIOD AND PREGNANCY. Appears safe in small amounts when breastfeeding.

Contraindications and precautions: Diabetes mellitus, haemorrhage, coagulation or haemorrhagic conditions. Do not confuse with Marsh marigold.

Adverse effects: Orally – nausea, vomiting, diarrhoea. Topically – skin irritation (rare).

Interactions: Therapeutic oral doses, prolonged, excessive or inappropriate use may interact with anticoagulants and antiplatelet drugs: heparin, warfarin, aspirin, enoxaparin. Also antidiabetic medication, lithium, oral drugs (may impair absorption). Anticoagulant herbs: angelica, clove, garlic, ginger, ginkgo, Panax ginseng, red clover, turmeric, willow. Hypoglycaemic herbs: bitter melon, chromium, devil's claw, fenugreek, garlic, guar gum, horse chestnut, Panax ginseng, psyllium, Siberian ginseng.

MARSH MARIGOLD
Caltha palustris, Caltha alba Herbal remedy.

Indications: Orally – for pain, cramps, dysmenorrhoea, as a laxative, diuretic, for bronchitis, jaundice, hepatobiliary disorders, arthritis, to lower cholesterol, raise blood sugar. Topically – for skin lesions and sores.

Safety in pregnancy: AVOID USE OF FRESH ABOVE-GROUND PARTS IN PREGNANCY. Safety of dried marigold or roots is unknown. Highly alkaloid toxins make marsh marigold unsafe for humans.

Contraindications and precautions: Do not confuse with Calendula, Marigold, Marshmallow or Cowslip.

Adverse effects: Orally – severe gastrointestinal and renal irritation. Topically – contact dermatitis, allergic reactions.

Interactions: None documented.

MEADOWSWEET
Filipendula ulmaria Herbal remedy.

Indications: Orally – for colds, bronchitis, heartburn, peptic ulcer, gout, cystitis. Has anti-inflammatory and analgesic properties similar to aspirin.

Safety in pregnancy: AVOID IN PREGNANCY unless under the supervision of a qualified medical herbalist – may stimulate uterine contractions. Salicylate content may contribute to bleeding including miscarriage, antepartum haemorrhage, excessive postnatal lochia, especially with retained products of conception. Long-term consumption of tea possibly unsafe due to high level of tannins.

Contraindications and precautions: Aspirin allergy, bleeding, haemorrhagic disorders, asthma. Tannin level may impair absorption of essential nutrients, drugs.

Adverse effects: Gastric bleeding, renal irritation, hypersensitivity, nausea and vomiting, tinnitus, due to salicylates. Flowers also contain phyto-heparin with anticoagulant properties, although this is neutralized by other chemicals when the whole plant is used. Salicylate toxicity can occur with excessive or prolonged use – dehydration, metabolic acidosis, hyperthermia, haemorrhage or coagulopathy, hypoglycaemia, convulsions.

Interactions: Therapeutic oral doses, prolonged, excessive or inappropriate use may interact with aspirin, anticoagulants: heparin, warfarin, aspirin, enoxaparin. Also non-steroidal anti-inflammatories: ibuprofen; and with narcotics. Anticoagulant herbs: angelica, clove, garlic, ginger, ginkgo, Panax ginseng, red clover, turmeric, willow.

MEHNDI *see* Henna

MELATONIN
N-Acetyl-5-Methoxytryptamine Naturally occurring hormone derived from serotonin, also produced synthetically.

Indications: Orally – for jet lag, insomnia, sleep disorders, substance use withdrawal, smoking cessation, endometriosis, polycystic ovary syndrome, seasonal affective disorder, fibromyalgia, migraine, irritable bowel syndrome, attention deficit-hyperactivity disorder, eczema, hypertension, athletic performance, infertility, menopause, pre- and postoperative recovery, contraception. Topically – protection against sunburn. Also available in homeopathic dilution for anger, forgetfulness, dyslexia, headache, irritability.

Safety in pregnancy: AVOID THERAPEUTIC ORAL DOSES AND PROLONGED USE IN PRE-CONCEPTION PERIOD – may inhibit ovulation. Caution: insufficient information on safety during pregnancy and when breastfeeding. Homeopathic dilution safe when used appropriately.

Contraindications and precautions: Do not drive or operate machinery for 4 to 6 hours after taking. Natural melatonin may be contaminated with viruses. Only available on prescription in the UK, European Union, Japan and Australia. Do not use homeopathic product prophylactically, or for prolonged periods, to avoid reverse proving.

Adverse effects: Orally – headache, dizziness, nausea, drowsiness, transient depressive symptoms, tremor, anxiety, abdominal cramps, irritability, reduced alertness, confusion or disorientation, hypotension. Prolonged or excessive use can lead to intractable insomnia.

Interactions: Therapeutic oral doses, prolonged, excessive or inappropriate use may interact with anticoagulants and antiplatelet drugs: heparin, warfarin, aspirin, enoxaparin. Also antidiabetic medication, anticonvulsants, alcohol, contraceptive Pill, theophylline, diazepam, phenytoin, imipramine, ondansetron, fentanyl, immunosuppressants. Anticoagulant herbs: angelica, clove, garlic, ginger, ginkgo, meadowsweet, Panax ginseng, red clover, turmeric, willow. Hypotensive herbs: cat's claw, coenzyme Q10, fish oil, L-arginine, stinging nettle. Sedative herbs: calamus, California poppy, catnip, hops, Jamaican dogwood, kava, St John's wort, skullcap, valerian, yerba mansa. Also caffeine, echinacea, hyssop oil, juniper, rosemary, sage, St John's wort, vitex agnus castus, wormwood.

MELISSA *see* Lemon balm

MILK THISTLE
Silybum marianum Herbal remedy.

Indications: Orally – for hangover, toxin-induced liver damage, alcohol-related liver disease, cirrhosis, hepatitis. Also for dysmenorrhoea, menopausal symptoms, lactation, fertility issues, indigestion, gall bladder disease, ulcerative colitis, diabetes mellitus, chemotherapy-induced nephrotoxicity, malaria, depression and other mental health disorders, multiple sclerosis. Topically – for radiation dermatitis.

Safety in pregnancy: Caution: little information available on safety. Animal research suggests increased risk of embryo resorption, intrauterine growth retardation, skeletal abnormalities, but no human evidence to date. Appears safe in small doses when breastfeeding; may promote lactation.

Contraindications and precautions: Diabetes mellitus, hormone-sensitive conditions – breast, uterine and ovarian cancer, endometriosis, fibroids. People with allergy to plants in the Asteraceae/Compositae family – ragweed, chrysanthemums, marigolds, daisies.

Adverse effects: Orally – diarrhoea, nausea, indigestion, flatulence, abdominal bloating. Occasionally, allergic reactions – pruritus, rash, urticaria, eczema, anaphylaxis.

Interactions: Therapeutic oral doses, prolonged, excessive or inappropriate use may interact with antidiabetic medication and anticoagulants: heparin, warfarin, aspirin, enoxaparin. Also pentazocine, propranolol, theophylline, diclofenac, amitriptyline, diazepam, metronidazole, tamoxifen, chlorpromazine, oestrogens, cimetidine, indinavir. Hypoglycaemic herbs: bitter melon, devil's claw, fenugreek, garlic, horse chestnut, Panax ginseng, psyllium, Siberian ginseng.

MISTLETOE, European
Viscum album Herbal remedy.

Indications: Orally – for cancer and reducing chemotherapy and radiation therapy side effects; for hypertension, haemorrhoids, epilepsy, infantile convulsions; depression, anxiety; insomnia, headache; amenorrhoea; menopausal symptoms.

Safety in pregnancy: AVOID IN PREGNANCY AND BREASTFEEDING – may be abortifacient, cause preterm labour, hypertonic uterine contractions, excessive lochia, especially if retained products of conception.

Contraindications and precautions: Hepatic and cardiac disease; autoimmune diseases.

Adverse effects: Orally – vomiting, diarrhoea, intestinal cramps, hepatitis, hypotension, anaphylactic reactions, constricted pupils, convulsions, coma, death. May interfere with liver function test results.

Interactions: Therapeutic oral doses, prolonged, excessive or inappropriate use may interact with antihypertensives, carbamazepine, isoniazid, tamoxifen, valproic acid, niacin, nitrofurantoin, immunosuppressants, corticosteroids. Hepatotoxic herbs: chaparral, comfrey, pennyroyal oil, red yeast. Hypotensive herbs: cat's claw, coenzyme Q10, fish oil, stinging nettle. Also hawthorn.

MONK'S HOOD *see* Aconite, herbal remedy

MOOSE ELM *see* Slippery elm

MOTHERWORT
Leonurus artemisia, Leonurus cardiaca Herbal remedy, also known as Common motherwort, Lion's tail. Also *Leonurus japonica*, Chinese motherwort, used interchangeably.

Indications: Orally – for dysmenorrhoea, menopausal symptoms, amenorrhoea, stress in pregnancy. Also for hypertension, heart arrhythmias, digestive disorders, cancer, alcohol withdrawal, insomnia. Topically – wounds, skin inflammation, itching and shingles. Intramuscularly or by intrauterine injection – postpartum haemorrhage, postoperative bleeding after Caesarean section, termination of pregnancy.

Safety in pregnancy: AVOID IN PREGNANCY, LABOUR, CAESAREAN SECTION AND TERMINATION OF PREGNANCY unless under the supervision of a qualified medical herbalist – inappropriate doses may cause miscarriage, preterm labour due to emmenagoguic alkaloids.

Contraindications and precautions: Hypotension, coagulation/haemorrhagic disorders, impending surgery. Avoid if allergic to other plants in the mint family. Do not confuse with *Leonotis nepetifolia* (Lion's ear, Wild or Klip dagga, a southern African emmenagoguic and purgative remedy, often smoked for recreational purposes).

Adverse effects: Orally – diarrhoea, stomach irritation, uterine bleeding, allergic reactions. Topically – contact dermatitis, photosensitivity (oil).

Interactions: Therapeutic oral doses, prolonged, excessive or inappropriate use may interact with central nervous system depressants. Anticoagulant and antiplatelet drugs and herbs: angelica, clove, fenugreek, feverfew, garlic, ginger, ginkgo, meadowsweet, Panax ginseng, poplar, red clover, turmeric, willow bark.

MUGWORT
Artemisia vulgaris Herbal remedy, Chinese energy technique.

Indications: Orally – for menstrual problems, irregular periods, to promote circulation. Also for abdominal colic, persistent vomiting, diarrhoea, constipation, to stimulate gastric juice and bile secretion, hysteria, convulsions in children, as a sedative. Topically – itching. In Chinese medicine, used in dried form as a heat source directed at a specific acupuncture point, for moxibustion to convert breech presentation to cephalic in third trimester; also for other conditions (non-pregnant).

Safety in pregnancy: AVOID ORAL HERBAL USE IN PREGNANCY – abortifacient, may cause miscarriage, preterm labour, fetal neurological damage. No information available on oral use during lactation. Dried for use as moxibustion – safe for breech presentation, subject to contraindications and precautions below.

Contraindications and precautions: Moxibustion for breech presentation – do not use before 34 weeks' gestation. Ensure purchase of *mild* moxibustion sticks with no other chemical additives. Check fetal presentation, estimated fetal size, maternal and fetal wellbeing prior to commencing treatment regimen. Contraindicated in women with previous Caesarean section uterine scar, especially if within previous two years. Avoid with multiple pregnancy, liquor volume irregularities, placenta praevia, fetal abnormalities, maternal hypertension, antepartum haemorrhage, diabetes mellitus. Contraindicated in women due for elective Caesarean section for medical or obstetric reason. Avoid with oblique or transverse lie, unstable lie, contracted pelvis, cephalopelvic disproportion. Avoid if external cephalic version contraindicated. Also avoid with asthma and hay fever; keep away from children (due to smoke from burning moxa). Do not allow burning moxa sticks to touch the skin. Moxibustion should only be performed by an appropriately qualified acupuncturist or Chinese medicine practitioner; midwives, doulas and doctors may advise but not normally perform a course of treatment (check indemnity insurance). Women should be discouraged from self-treatment unless under the supervision of a practitioner who has assessed the woman as medically suited to moxibustion. Course of treatment should be completed to ensure further descent of the fetal head. Moxibustion for reasons other than breech presentation – only under the supervision of an appropriately experienced acupuncturist.

Adverse effects: Moxibustion for breech presentation – respiratory sensitivity, exacerbation of hay fever, asthma, nausea, headache; failure of breech to convert to cephalic presentation. Theoretically, continuation of treatment in the event of cephalopelvic disproportion could lead to extension of the fetal head into brow or face presentation. Herbal use, orally – respiratory reactions; topically – contact dermatitis.

Interactions: No interactions with drugs documented. Herbs: allergic reaction from oral use if sensitive to plants in the Asteraceae/Compositae family – ragweed, chrysanthemum, marigold, daisies. Allergic reactions possible if sensitive to birch, celery, wild carrot, and also, theoretically, to honey, royal jelly, hazelnut, olive, latex, peach, kiwi, sage. Strong odour from moxibustion to turn breech presentation may inactivate homeopathic remedies.

MUPFUTA *see* Castor oil

NATRUM MUR

Natrum muriaticum Homeopathic remedy, tissue salt from sodium chloride, also called Nat mur.

Obstetric indications: Failure to progress in labour; heartburn; backache; headaches; grief. Sometimes used to correct breech presentation.

Key features: Dryness and extreme thirst. Excessive perspiration and mucous discharge; vagina dry but leucorrhoea watery, like raw egg white. Symptoms triggered by intense emotions – grief, embarrassment, anger, fright. Labour contractions – pulsating; tearing, stitching, jerking, pressing, burning. Breech presentation with "fluid" issues – either excessive as with oedema, diarrhoea, rhinitis, polyhydramnios or inadequate as with dry skin, hair, constipation, oligohydramnios.

Emotional symptoms: Dwells on past unpleasant experiences; hopeless about future; moods fluctuate from fear or sadness to inappropriate laughter. Wants to be alone but feels forsaken and unlovable. Masks emotional vulnerability; easily angered, offended. Vivid dreams of robbers. Inhibition – difficulty passing urine in public toilets.

Better for: Lying down; fasting; perspiring; fresh air; firm pressure.

Worse for: Consolation; sun; before menstruation; mental exertion; between 1000–1100 hours; having to engage in conversation; fats; bread.

Safety: Do not use for breech presentation with oligo- or polyhydramnios unless under the supervision of a qualified homeopath. Do not use if there are any medical or obstetric complications. Not to be used as a replacement for standard medical care. Do not use with aromatherapy essential oils, topically or by inhalation, or with antacids, decongestants, laxatives or cough lozenges – inactivates the remedy. Do not take with food or drink. Do not take prophylactically – may lead to reverse proving. Should not be used by women who do not fit the symptom picture to avoid reverse proving. To be handled by the intended recipient only.

NDOVE YENZOU *see* Elephant dung

NEROLI

Citrus aurantium Essential oil, also known as Orange blossom.

Indications: Topically – essential oil used in aromatherapy for relaxation, anxiety, fear, depression, pain relief in labour, to enhance mood, as an aphrodisiac, for insomnia, nausea, constipation, diarrhoea, to reduce blood pressure, for wound healing, skin care, to reduce striae gravidarum; antibacterial, antiviral, antispasmodic.

Safety in pregnancy: Essential oil used in aromatherapy appears safe in doses up to 1.5% in pregnancy and 2% in labour and postnatal period.

Contraindications and precautions: Essential oil, topically or by inhalation – avoid with allergy to citrus fruit; caution with hay fever triggered by flower pollens – may have psychosomatic effect. Avoid exposure of skin to direct sunlight for at least 2 hours – risk of photosensitivity. Do not ingest. Do not use neat on skin or directly in a birthing pool. Use a diffuser for a maximum of 15–20 minutes in any hour; do not vaporize in the second stage of labour to avoid neonatal exposure; do not diffuse near neonates, elderly, ill people or those allergic to citrus fruit. Do not diffuse near animals – toxic to cats and dogs. Do not diffuse in public areas or in excessive amounts which spread to public areas of maternity unit, to avoid excessive exposure of the woman, baby, visitors and staff to potential adverse effects. Discontinue use if any allergic reactions occur to avoid accumulative reaction to specific chemicals – may lead to anaphylactic shock in severe cases. Do not use with or store near homeopathic remedies. Store in a refrigerator to avoid rapid oxidation – shelf life of 3–6 months. Do not confuse with Sweet orange or Bitter orange.

Adverse effects: Photosensitivity; asthma or hay fever attack triggered by psychosomatic effect of aroma.

Interactions: Topically – prolonged, excessive or inappropriate use may theoretically interact with anticoagulants and antiplatelet drugs: heparin, warfarin, aspirin, diclofenac, ibuprofen, enoxaparin. Anticoagulant herbs: angelica, clove, fenugreek, feverfew, garlic, ginger, ginkgo, Panax ginseng, poplar, red clover, turmeric.

NERVE ROOT

Cypripedium pubescens Herbal remedy, also known as Lady's slipper, American valerian.

Indications: Orally – for menorrhagia, to prevent miscarriage, diarrhoea, insomnia; emotional tension; hysteria; anxiety. Topically – for vaginal pruritus. Also available in homeopathic dilution for skin symptoms, similar in character to Rhus toxicodendron, and for headache and emotional problems.

Safety in pregnancy: Homeopathic remedy appears safe when used under the supervision of a qualified homeopath. AVOID HERBAL PREPARATION IN PREGNANCY unless under the supervision of a qualified medical herbalist. Caution: insufficient information on safety when breastfeeding.

Contraindications and precautions: Avoid herbal remedy with pethidine, morphine. Advise women not to self-medicate with homeopathic preparation to avoid reverse proving. Member of the orchid family, an endangered species in some areas. Do not confuse with Valerian or with *Cypripedium parviflorum*, also known as Lady's slipper.

Adverse effects: Dermatitis, restlessness, hallucinations.

Interactions: Possible interactions with pethidine, other hallucinatory analgesics.

NIGELLA
Nigella sativa Herbal remedy, also known as Black seed.

Indications: Orally – to promote menstruation, for contraception, menopausal symptoms, mastalgia, lactation, male infertility. Also for colic, heartburn, diarrhoea, constipation, haemorrhoids, ulcerative colitis, *Helicobacter pylori* infection, asthma, respiratory conditions, hypertension, opioid withdrawal, to improve cognitive function. Topically – for headache, skin conditions, nasal dryness, osteoarthritis, rheumatism. Intravaginally – to treat fungal infection.

Safety in pregnancy: Appears safe in amounts commonly used in foods. AVOID THERAPEUTIC ORAL DOSES AND INTRAVAGINAL USE IN PRECONCEPTION PERIOD, PREGNANCY AND LABOUR – may affect embryonic implantation, affect uterine muscle in pregnancy, either as a relaxant or stimulant, increasing the risk of miscarriage. May decrease/inhibit uterine contractions in labour. Appears safe when breastfeeding in small amounts.

Contraindications and precautions: Avoid with epilepsy, diabetes mellitus, hypo- or hypertension, especially if on medication.

Adverse effects: Orally and topically – skin itching. Orally – constipation, abdominal discomfort, nausea, vomiting. May exacerbate convulsions in those with epilepsy. Hypoglycaemia, hypotension.

Interactions: Therapeutic oral doses, prolonged, excessive or inappropriate use may interact with anticoagulants and antiplatelet drugs: heparin, warfarin, aspirin, diclofenac, ibuprofen, enoxaparin. Also antidiabetic medication, antihypertensives, diuretics. Herbs: angelica, California poppy, catnip, cat's claw, clove, coenzyme Q10, devil's claw, fenugreek, garlic, ginger, ginkgo, hops, horse chestnut, Jamaican dogwood, kava, Panax ginseng, psyllium, St John's wort, Siberian ginseng, skullcap, stinging nettle, valerian, yerba mansa.

NUTMEG
Myristica fragrans Herbal remedy.

Indications: Orally – diarrhoea, nausea, colic, flatulence, insomnia, to promote menstrual flow, induce miscarriage, as hallucinogen, general tonic. Topically – essential oil used as an analgesic, especially for mouth sores, toothache. Nutmeg derived from shelled, dried seed; mace derived from seed husk.

Safety in pregnancy: Caution with excessive consumption in foods during pregnancy. AVOID ORAL, TOPICAL AND INHALATIONAL USE IN

PRECONCEPTION PERIOD, PREGNANCY AND LABOUR – safrole content may be mutagenic, abortifacient, carcinogenic, hepatotoxic. May have unpredictable effects on labour contractions, possibly leading to fetal distress, hypertonic uterine action. Advise caution: no information on safety of therapeutic doses or essential oil when breastfeeding.

Contraindications and precautions: Avoid herbal remedy and essential oil with sub-fertility, may affect implantation. Do not use for pain relief in labour or post-Caesarean section.

Adverse effects: Overdose can cause severe cardiovascular, gastrointestinal, muscular, neurological adverse effects. Myristicin content is hallucinogenic and psychotropic – excessive use can be fatal.

Interactions: Therapeutic oral doses, prolonged, excessive or inappropriate use may interact with pethidine, morphine, anticholinergic drugs, cerebral nervous system depressants, monoamine oxidase inhibitors. Herbs with sedative effects: calamus, California poppy, catnip, hops, Jamaican dogwood, kava, St John's wort, skullcap, valerian, yerba mansa. Potentially toxic herbs containing safrole: basil, camphor, cinnamon.

NUX VOMICA

Strychnos nux-vomica Homeopathic remedy from poison nut tree (strychnine).

Obstetric indications: Constipation with backache, ineffectual urges to empty bowel, feeling of incomplete emptying. Nausea – feels vomiting would relieve symptoms, sour, bitter belching and retching. Does not want to face labour. Contractions weak, spasms in back extending to thigh; urge to defecate during contractions. Pain – pulsating, tearing, stitching, sharp. Also for common cold, influenza; common remedy for over-indulgence in food, alcohol, tobacco, drugs.

Key features: Hangover-like symptoms – fragile head after excessive eating or drinking; headache like nail driven into forehead; abdominal discomfort – like a stone in the base of the stomach, with indigestion, flatulence; vertigo; insomnia; craves fatty highly seasoned foods. Often called "man's remedy" – opposite profile to homeopathic Pulsatilla.

Emotional symptoms: Irritable, impatient, angry, quarrelsome, critical. Typical workaholic personality, perfectionist, highly charged, stimulant-driven lifestyle. Desires privacy, music irritates.

Better for: Warmth; rest; firm pressure; evening; damp weather; being alone; washing.

Worse for: Noise; cold; touch; spicy food; stimulants, dry conditions; between 0300–0400 hours; mental exertion.

Safety: Do not confuse with poison nut, herbal remedy – contains toxic strychnine, fatal even in moderate amounts. Do not use if there are any medical or obstetric complications. Not to be used as a replacement for standard medical care. Do not use with aromatherapy essential oils, topically or by inhalation, or with antacids, decongestants, laxatives or cough lozenges – inactivates the remedy. Do not take with food or drink. Do not take prophylactically – may lead to reverse proving. Should not be used by women who do not fit the symptom picture to avoid reverse proving. To be handled by the intended recipient only.

NZU *see* **Calabash chalk**

OAK MOSS
Evernia prunastri Herbal remedy.

Indications: Orally – as gastrointestinal tonic.

Safety in pregnancy: Appears safe when taken orally as a tea for short periods. AVOID THERAPEUTIC ORAL DOSES, PROLONGED OR EXCESSIVE CONSUMPTION OF TEA IN PREGNANCY – contains thujone in small amounts, can cause miscarriage.

Contraindications and precautions: Do not confuse with tree moss.

Adverse effects: Orally – restlessness, vomiting, vertigo, renal toxicity, convulsions, possible allergic reactions. Topically – contact dermatitis, especially if allergic to lichen and other moss types.

Interactions: Therapeutic oral doses, prolonged, excessive or inappropriate use may interact with thujone-containing herbs: sage, tansy, thuja (cedar), tree moss, wormwood.

OLIBANUM *see* **Frankincense**

OLIVE OIL
Olea europaea Herbal remedy.

Indications: Orally – for hypertension, hypercholesterolaemia, obesity, diabetes mellitus, breast and ovarian cancer, migraine headache, gallstones, constipation, *Helicobacter pylori* infection. Leaf traditionally used orally for influenza, common cold, pneumonia, herpes, shingles, HIV/AIDS, chronic fatigue; various serious infections; as a diuretic and antipyretic. Topically – for tinnitus, earache, lice, wounds, burns, skin conditions including striae gravidarum, ultraviolet damage. Also used as carrier oil for massage.

Safety in pregnancy: Appears safe in amounts commonly used in foods. Caution with dermal use, may block pores, damage skin cells. Thick consistency, distinctive aroma – not generally appropriate for aromatherapy use.

Contraindications and precautions: Do not use as massage oil for babies – may damage naturally protective fatty skin cells and increase risk of childhood eczema.

Adverse effects: Topically – contact dermatitis.

Interactions: Therapeutic oral doses, prolonged, excessive or inappropriate use may interact with anticoagulants and antiplatelet drugs: heparin, warfarin, aspirin, diclofenac, ibuprofen, enoxaparin. Also antidiabetic medication, antihypertensives. Herbs: angelica, cat's claw, clove, coenzyme Q10, devil's claw, fenugreek, garlic, ginger, ginkgo, horse chestnut, Panax ginseng, psyllium, red clover, Siberian ginseng, stinging nettle, turmeric, willow.

ORANGE BLOSSOM *see* Neroli

ORANGE, Bitter

Citrus aurantium, Citrus bigarradia Herbal remedy.

Indications: Orally – to regulate appetite, for heartburn, flatulence, duodenal ulcer, constipation, diarrhoea, weight loss; for nasal congestion, allergic rhinitis, insomnia, anxiety, to regulate blood lipids, blood sugar, mineral metabolism, for prolapse of uterus, anus, rectum. Topically – for skin inflammation, conjunctival irritation, muscular pain, bruises, phlebitis. Topically, essential oil in aromatherapy – as an analgesic, for premenstrual syndrome, digestive disturbance. Used in Ayurvedic medicine as an aid to relaxation.

Safety in pregnancy: Appears safe in amounts commonly used in foods. AVOID ORAL THERAPEUTIC DOSES IN PREGNANCY. Topically, essential oil in aromatherapy – minimize doses to 0.5% in pregnancy, 1% in labour and postnatally – risk of photosensitivity.

Contraindications and precautions: Essential oil in aromatherapy – avoid in women who are allergic to citrus fruit. Avoid exposure of skin to direct sunlight for at least 2 hours after topical use; discontinue if skin is itching. Do not ingest. Do not use neat on skin or directly in a birthing pool. Do not apply directly to breasts in postnatal period, or wash with water before the baby starts feeding to avoid adverse neonatal effects from ingestion. Use a diffuser for a maximum of 15–20 minutes in any hour; do not vaporize in the second stage of labour to avoid neonatal exposure. Do not diffuse near neonates, the elderly, ill people and those who are allergic to citrus fruit or animals. Do not diffuse in public areas or use excessive amounts that spread to public areas of a maternity unit, to avoid excessive exposure of the woman, baby, visitors and staff to potential adverse effects. Discontinue use if any allergic reactions occur to avoid accumulative reaction to specific chemicals – may lead to anaphylactic shock in severe cases. Store in a refrigerator to avoid rapid oxidation. Avoid prolonged use – furanocoumarins may cause malignant skin changes. Do not use with or store near homeopathic remedies. Orally – avoid with diabetes mellitus, hypertension, certain types of glaucoma, prior to surgery. Do not confuse with Sweet orange.

Adverse effects: Therapeutic oral doses – diarrhoea, flatulence. Excessive, prolonged or inappropriate use – synephrine content (similar to Ephedra) may cause vasoconstriction leading to headaches, tachycardia, hypertension, cardiac arrest, syncope, angina, myocardial infarction, ventricular arrhythmia, death. Topically – photosensitivity, skin irritation.

Interactions: Therapeutic oral doses, prolonged, excessive or inappropriate use may interact with monoamine oxidase inhibitors, antidiabetic medication, caffeine, fluoxetine. Stimulant herbs: black tea, cola nut, ma huang, oolong tea. Caffeine. Panax ginseng may cause cardiac arrhythmia.

ORANGE, Sweet

Citrus X sinensis Essential oil.

Indications: Topically or by inhalation, essential oil in aromatherapy – for relaxation, mood enhancing, pain relief, constipation, aids circulation, oedema, may aid smooth muscle contraction, skin care, may aid lymphatic drainage; antibacterial, antifungal, antiseptic. Orally – fruit and peel used for hypertension, renal calculi, raised cholesterol, gastrointestinal conditions.

Safety in pregnancy: Topically and by inhalation, essential oil safe in doses up to 1.5% in pregnancy and 2% in labour and postnatal period. Orally – appears safe in amounts commonly used in foods.

Contraindications and precautions: Orally, topically and by inhalation – avoid in women who are allergic to citrus fruit. Essential oil, topically or by inhalation – avoid exposure of skin to direct sunlight for at least 2 hours after topical use; discontinue if skin itching. Do not ingest. Do not use neat on skin or directly in a birthing pool. Use a diffuser for a maximum of 15–20 minutes in any hour; do not vaporize in the second stage of labour to avoid neonatal exposure; do not diffuse near neonates, elderly, ill people or those who are allergic to citrus fruit. Do not diffuse near animals – toxic to cats and dogs. Do not diffuse in public areas or use excessive amounts which spread to public areas of maternity unit, to avoid excessive exposure of the woman, baby, visitors and staff to potential adverse effects. Discontinue use if any allergic reactions occur to avoid accumulative reaction to specific chemicals – may lead to anaphylactic shock in severe cases. Store in a refrigerator to avoid rapid oxidization; shelf life of 3–6 months. Do not use with or store near homeopathic remedies. Do not confuse with Bitter orange.

Adverse effects: Topically – itching, photosensitivity. Orally – diarrhoea, flatulence.

Interactions: Therapeutic oral doses may interact with anticoagulants and antiplatelet drugs: heparin, warfarin, aspirin, diclofenac, ibuprofen, enoxaparin. Also certain antihypertensives, statins, antihistamine agents, certain antibiotics. Anticoagulant herbs: angelica, garlic, ginger, ginkgo, meadowsweet, Panax ginseng, turmeric, willow bark.

OREGANO

Origanum vulgare Herbal remedy, also known as Wild marjoram.

Indications: Orally – for common cold, influenza, cough, asthma, sinusitis, bronchitis; abdominal bloating, heartburn, dysmenorrhoea, urinary tract infection, headaches. Also for diabetes mellitus, bleeding after dental extraction. Topically – acne, athlete's foot, dandruff, gum disease, toothache, skin conditions, varicose veins, wounds, as an insect repellent.

Safety in pregnancy: Appears safe in amounts commonly used in foods. AVOID THERAPEUTIC ORAL DOSES AND TOPICAL USE OF ESSENTIAL OIL IN PREGNANCY – possible abortifacient and emmenagoguic effects.

Contraindications and precautions: Avoid in those allergic to thyme, basil, hyssop, lavender, marjoram, mint, sage. Avoid postnatally, if retained products of conception, due to emmenagoguic effect. Do not confuse with Marjoram.

Adverse effects: Oral and topical – skin irritation and allergy due to thymol content. Excessive oral use – nausea, vomiting, diarrhoea.

Interactions: Therapeutic oral doses, prolonged, excessive or inappropriate use may interact with anticoagulants and antiplatelet drugs: heparin, warfarin, aspirin, diclofenac, ibuprofen, enoxaparin. Also antidiabetic medication. Herbs: angelica, bitter melon, chromium, clove, devil's claw, fenugreek, garlic, ginger, ginkgo, horse chestnut, Panax ginseng, psyllium, red clover, Siberian ginseng, turmeric. May impair iron, zinc, copper absorption from food.

PALM DATES *see* Date palm

PANAX GINSENG *see* Ginseng

PAPAYA
Carica papaya Herbal remedy, also known as Pawpaw.

Indications: Orally – popular food to initiate labour contractions to avoid induction – papain thought to act similarly to Bromelain in pineapple. Orally in therapeutic doses – for gastrointestinal disorders, as a diuretic, for intestinal parasites, dengue fever, ageing skin, diabetes mellitus, to prevent human papilloma virus. Topically – for mouth inflammation and bleeding, wound healing, post-herpetic neuralgia.

Safety in pregnancy: AVOID EXCESSIVE CONSUMPTION IN PREGNANCY UNTIL TERM – considered "forbidden fruit" in pregnancy in the Middle East – may cause miscarriage if consumed in excessive amounts. Papaya contains papain, in particularly large amounts when fruit is green. Papain may be toxic to embryological development; may cause uterine contractions, leading to miscarriage, preterm labour.

Contraindications and precautions: Avoid at term if booked for elective Caesarean section – theoretical risk of excess bleeding. Avoid if allergic to latex, figs or kiwifruit – papain may increase risk of hypersensitivity reactions. Avoid with thyroid disorder – papain may exacerbate hypothyroidism or interfere with medication. Avoid oral and topical use with oesophageal trauma or duodenal ulcers – risk of perforation.

Adverse effects: Orally – skin irritation, allergic reactions – watery eyes, sneezing, cough, rhinitis. Excessive consumption in susceptible women could lead to anaphylaxis. Hypoglycaemia can develop from prolonged ingestion of fermented papaya.

Interactions: Therapeutic oral doses, prolonged, excessive or inappropriate use may interact with anticoagulants and antiplatelet drugs: heparin, warfarin, aspirin, diclofenac, ibuprofen, enoxaparin. Also antidiabetic medication, certain thyroid drugs. May interfere with urine-based tests for cannabinoids. Herbs: angelica, clove, devil's claw, fenugreek, feverfew, garlic, ginger, ginkgo, meadowsweet, Panax ginseng, poplar, red clover, turmeric, willow bark.

PARSLEY

Petroselinum crispum, Apium Petroselinum Herbal remedy.

Indications: Orally – to promote menstruation, reduce premenstrual oedema and congestion, induce miscarriage, as an aphrodisiac. Also for urinary tract infections, as a diuretic, for constipation, indigestion, cough, asthma, anaemia, hypertension, prostate and spleen conditions, as a breath freshener. Topically – for cracked or chapped skin, bruises, insect bites, lice, parasites, to stimulate hair growth.

Safety in pregnancy: AVOID THERAPEUTIC ORAL DOSES AND TOPICAL USE OF ESSENTIAL OIL IN PRECONCEPTION PERIOD AND PREGNANCY – contains high levels of apiole (parsley camphor), may cause miscarriage, renal and liver toxicity. Some commercial products containing parsley and Dong quai have been shown to cause congenital malformations.

Contraindications and precautions: Avoid large amounts in diet (over 200g). Avoid with any haemorrhagic/coagulation disorders. Beware diuretic effect. Note: Apiole is also found in celery leaf – avoid in pregnancy.

Adverse effects: Topically – photosensitivity, skin rash and irritation. Orally – ingestion of over 10g apiole may cause haemolytic anaemia, thrombocytopenia purpura, nephrosis, hepatic dysfunction, kidney irritation. Myristicin content can cause deafness, dizziness, hallucinations, hypotension, bradycardia, paralysis, hepatic and renal toxicity.

Interactions: Therapeutic oral doses, prolonged, excessive or inappropriate use may interact with anticoagulants and antiplatelet drugs: heparin, warfarin, aspirin, diclofenac, ibuprofen, enoxaparin. Also antidiabetic medication, amitriptyline, ondansetron, diuretics, sedatives, barbiturates. Herbs: angelica, clove, devil's claw, fenugreek, feverfew, garlic, ginger, ginkgo, guar gum, Panax ginseng, red clover, Siberian ginseng, turmeric.

PARTRIDGE BERRY *see* Squaw vine

PASQUE FLOWER *see* Pulsatilla

PASSIFLORA

Passiflora incarnata Herbal remedy, also known as Passionflower.

Indications: Orally – for menopausal symptoms, dysmenorrhoea, premenstrual syndrome. Also for insomnia, stress, pre-operative anxiety, diarrhoea, heartburn, pain relief, muscle cramps, asthma, opioid withdrawal symptoms. Topically – for haemorrhoids, burns, inflammation.

Safety in pregnancy: Appears safe in amounts commonly found in foods. AVOID THERAPEUTIC ORAL DOSES IN PRECONCEPTION PERIOD AND PREGNANCY – harmaline and harmine constituents may theoretically contribute to uterine stimulation leading to miscarriage, preterm labour, preterm membrane rupture, meconium aspiration syndrome.

Contraindications and precautions: Avoid with surgery – central nervous system effects may cause central nervous system depression when combined with anaesthetics.

Adverse effects: Orally – dizziness, confusion, drowsiness, muscle relaxation, allergy symptoms, uterine contractions, nosebleeds. Certain types of passiflora may contain hepatotoxic cyanogenic glycosides.

Interactions: Therapeutic oral doses, prolonged, excessive or inappropriate use may interact with lorazepam and other barbiturates, anaesthetics. Sedative herbs: California poppy, catnip, hops, Jamaican dogwood, kava, St John's wort, skullcap, valerian, yerba mansa.

PASSIONFLOWER *see* Passiflora

PAWPAW *see* Papaya

PELARGONIUM *see* Geranium

PENNYROYAL

Mentha pulegium, Pulegium vulgare Herbal remedy.

Indications: Orally – as abortifacient, to regulate menstrual cycle; as an antispasmodic, stimulant, diuretic. Also for common cold, gastrointestinal disorders, hepatobiliary disorders. Topically – essential oil used as an antiseptic, insect repellent, for skin diseases, gout, venomous bites, mouth sores and to kill fleas.

Safety in pregnancy: AVOID ORAL AND TOPICAL USE COMPLETELY IN PRECONCEPTION, ANTENATAL, INTRAPARTUM AND POSTNATAL PERIOD – highly toxic, can be fatal.

Contraindications and precautions: Member of the mint family: do not confuse with Peppermint (*Mentha piperata*) or spearmint (*Mentha spicata*).

Adverse effects: Orally – abdominal pain, nausea, vomiting, haematemesis, delirium, convulsions, disseminated intravascular coagulation, hepatic, renal and respiratory failure, death. Topically – urticarial rash, dermatitis.

Interactions: No specific interactions reported, but may decrease iron absorption.

PEPPERMINT
Mentha piperata Herbal remedy.

Indications: Orally – as tea from fresh leaves, for nausea, vomiting, diarrhoea, irritable bowel syndrome, heartburn and indigestion, flatulence, pregnancy sickness, dysmenorrhoea, menopausal hot flushes, abdominal cramps, headache, as a stimulant. Topically, essential oil in aromatherapy – for pregnancy, intrapartum, postoperative sickness, constipation, diarrhoea, irritable bowel syndrome, pain relief in pregnancy and labour, headache, breast engorgement, mood enhancer, circulatory stimulant; antibacterial, antifungal, anti-inflammatory, antispasmodic, antipruritic. By inhalation – for cough, common cold, sinusitis, pain relief, to improve cognitive function, stress.

Safety in pregnancy: Orally – appears safe in pregnancy in amounts commonly found in foods. Tea not safe for babies and infants – menthol content can cause choking sensation. Topically – essential oil used in aromatherapy is safe in doses up to 1.5% in pregnancy and 2% in labour. Controversy over use in postnatal period thought to reduce milk supply – advice is to avoid if lactation is poor.

Contraindications and precautions: Avoid oral and topical use with cardiac disease, especially antenatal inpatients; also epilepsy, glucose 6 phosphate dehydrogenase (G6PD) disease, gall bladder problems. Orally, peppermint tea – do not use for sickness with accompanying heartburn. Essential oil – do not ingest unless medically prescribed, usually as enteric-coated capsules or diluted peppermint water. Essential oil, topically or by inhalation – do not use on or vaporize near neonates, infants or young children – may exacerbate physiological jaundice; excessive amounts can cause reflex apnoea. Do not use neat on skin or directly in a birthing pool. Use a diffuser for a maximum of 15–20 minutes in any hour; do not vaporize in the second stage of labour to avoid neonatal exposure; do not diffuse near neonates, elderly or ill people. Do not diffuse near animals – toxic to cats and dogs. Do not diffuse in public areas or use excessive amounts which spread to public areas of maternity unit, to avoid excessive exposure of the woman, baby, visitors and staff to potential adverse effects. If lactation adequate and essential oil chosen for topical use in postnatal period, maximum dose 2%; do not diffuse near the baby and do not apply directly to the breasts. Discontinue use if any allergic reactions occur to avoid accumulative reaction to specific chemicals – may lead to anaphylactic shock in severe cases. Do not use with or store near homeopathic remedies. Store in a refrigerator to avoid rapid oxidation.

Adverse effects: Orally, including excessive consumption of tea – heartburn, nausea, vomiting, anal or perianal burning, abdominal pain, belching, dry mouth, diarrhoea, increased appetite, blurred vision. May be hepatotoxic or neurotoxic in large doses. Topically, essential oil in aromatherapy – allergic reactions, skin irritation, burning, erythema, contact dermatitis, especially if used neat. Excessive or prolonged topical or oral use, including tea, may lead to insomnia, mental stimulation and sleep disturbance, interfere with iron absorption, cause palpitations. Peppermint leaf orally in therapeutic doses may interfere with hormone test results.

Interactions: Therapeutic oral doses, prolonged, excessive or inappropriate use may interact with anticoagulants and antiplatelet drugs: heparin, warfarin, aspirin, diclofenac, ibuprofen, enoxaparin. Also antacids, cimetidine, ranitidine, cyclosporine, amitriptyline, ondansetron, propranolol, theophylline, verapamil, diazepam. Anticoagulant herbs: angelica, clove, fenugreek, feverfew, garlic, ginger, ginkgo, Panax ginseng, poplar, red clover, turmeric.

PHYTOLACCA

Phytolacca decandra Homeopathic remedy from poke root.

Obstetric indications: Breast engorgement; mastitis; breast abscess; cracked, sore nipples. Also for glandular fever; mumps; tonsillitis.

Key features: Disorders of glandular tissue; especially mammary glands; restlessness, exhaustion; electric shooting pains. Copious saliva with metallic taste; bruised sensation all over the body; vertigo with dimness of vision. Breasts – hard, hot, inflamed, purplish hue on left side; spasmodic intolerable pain radiating through whole body when feeding.

Emotional symptoms: Irritable; worn out, indifferent to life, herself and work; feels will die, gives up.

Better for: Warmth; open air; dry weather; rest; lying on affected side; cold drinks.

Worse for: Cold, damp conditions; rising from bed; starting to move; prolonged activity; hot drinks; when baby suckles; swallowing; night-time.

Safety: Do not use if there are any medical or obstetric complications. Not to be used as a replacement for standard medical care. Do not use with aromatherapy essential oils, topically or by inhalation, or with antacids, decongestants, laxatives or cough lozenges – inactivates the remedy. Do not take with food or drink. Do not take prophylactically – may lead to reverse proving. Should not be used by women who do not fit the symptom picture to avoid reverse proving. To be handled by the intended recipient only. Do not confuse with herbal Poke root.

PINEAPPLE *see* Bromelain

PLANTAIN, Great
Plantago major, *Plantago asiatica* Herbal remedy.

Indications: Orally – for cystitis with haematuria, bronchitis, colds, bleeding haemorrhoids, antiseptic, anti-inflammatory, antibacterial. Topically – for skin conditions, eye irritation.

Safety in pregnancy: AVOID THERAPEUTIC DOSES IN PREGNANCY – may affect uterine tone, theoretical risk of miscarriage, preterm labour.

Contraindications and precautions: Avoid confusion with buckhorn plantain (*Plantago lanceolata*), Blond psyllium (*Plantago ovata*) and black psyllium (*Plantago psyllium*).

Adverse effects: Orally – diarrhoea, hypotension. May interfere with clotting factors due to vitamin K content. Topically – allergic contact dermatitis. Avoid in people allergic to melons or with known plantain sensitivity.

Interactions: Therapeutic oral doses, prolonged, excessive or inappropriate use may interact with anticoagulants and antiplatelet drugs: heparin, warfarin, aspirin, diclofenac, ibuprofen, enoxaparin. Anticoagulant herbs: angelica, clove, fenugreek, feverfew, garlic, ginger, ginkgo, meadowsweet, Panax ginseng, poplar, red clover, turmeric, willow bark.

POISON GOOSEBERRY *see* Ashwagandha

POISON NUT *see* Nux vomica

POKE ROOT
Phytolacca americana, *Phytolacca decandra* Herbal remedy, also called pokeweed.

Indications: Orally – for dysmenorrhoea, mastitis, breast abscess. Also for respiratory tract inflammation and infections, skin infections, to induce vomiting. Topically – for skin conditions, bruises, sprains, inflammation, oedema.

Safety in pregnancy: AVOID ORAL AND TOPICAL USE IN PREGNANCY – all parts of the plant are toxic, even in small amounts, may have uterine stimulant and abortifacient effects.

Contraindications and precautions: Unsafe for any medicinal use. Do not confuse with homeopathic Phytolacca.

Adverse effects: Nausea, vomiting, cramping, abdominal pain, diarrhoea, burning mouth and throat, hypotension, haematemesis, tachycardia, respiratory failure, urinary incontinence, haematological changes, convulsions, death.

Interactions: None documented.

PSYLLIUM

Plantago arenaria Herbal remedy.

Indications: Orally – for chronic constipation, to soften stools with haemorrhoids, for diarrhoea, irritable bowel syndrome, other gastrointestinal symptoms. Also for anal fissures, anorectal surgery, elevated cholesterol.

Safety in pregnancy: Safe enough in moderate oral doses, but advise adequate fluid intake to avoid choking and oesophageal obstruction.

Contraindications and precautions: Avoid with diabetes mellitus, swallowing, gastrointestinal and oesophageal disorders, known hypersensitivity to psyllium. Do not confuse with Blond psyllium, buckhorn plantain, great plantain, water plantain.

Adverse effects: Flatulence, bloating, diarrhoea. Gastrointestinal obstruction if taken with insufficient fluids. Hypoglycaemia. May impair absorption of essential nutrients, for example as calcium, copper, magnesium, iron, zinc, sodium, potassium – caution with deficiency symptoms.

Interactions: Therapeutic oral doses, prolonged, excessive or inappropriate use may interact with antidiabetic medication, carbamazepine, lithium. Also with other drugs taken by mouth – impaired absorption. Herbs: devil's claw, fenugreek, Panax ginseng, Siberian ginseng.

PULSATILLA

Pulsatilla nigricans Homeopathic remedy from Wind flower, also known as Pasque flower.

Obstetric indications: Pain, failure to progress; postnatal afterpains; constipation; leg or vulval varicosities and haemorrhoids. Popular remedy for correcting malposition, unstable (changeable) lie, breech presentation. Also for indecisiveness about options in pregnancy, labour. Labour contractions weak, short, intermittent, changeable.

Key features: Erratic, changeable symptoms – bowels, menstruation, fetal position or presentation, pain, generally more noticeable on the right side. Dry mucous membranes, coated tongue with lack of thirst. Craves indigestible foods, fresh air. Fear of dogs; weird dreams. May sleep on abdomen or with hands above head. Hypotension, with vertigo when looking upwards; prone to anaemia, varicose veins. Often called "woman's remedy" – opposite profile to homeopathic Nux vomica.

Emotional symptoms: Indecisive, changeable moods; affectionate; desires company; sulky, easily persuaded, easily offended; tearful when talking – sympathetic to others' problems and tends to think emotionally; shy; child-like; fear of being alone, dark, own sanity.

Better for: Continued or gentle motion; fresh air; cold applications; crying; sympathy; cold drinks; touch.

Worse for: Getting heated; warm, stuffy atmosphere; rich food, pork; puberty; menstruation; evening and during the night.

Safety: Do not use with standard iron therapy for anaemia, and consult a qualified homeopath. Do not use if there are any medical or obstetric complications. Not to be used as a replacement for standard medical care. Do not use with aromatherapy essential oils, topically or by inhalation, or with antacids, decongestants, laxatives or cough lozenges – inactivates the remedy. Do not take with food or drink. Do not take prophylactically – may lead to reverse proving. Should not be used by women who do not fit the symptom picture to avoid reverse proving. To be handled by the intended recipient only. Do not confuse with Pulsatilla (Wind flower, Pasque flower), herbal remedy.

RAGWORT

Senecio vulgaris, *Senecio jacobaea* Herbal remedy, also known as Alpine ragwort, Tansy ragwort, Stinking willie.

Indications: Orally – to induce menstruation, for wound healing, constipation, colic, to induce sweating, to detoxify. Topically – for muscle and joint pain.

Safety in pregnancy: AVOID ORAL AND TOPICAL USE IN PREGNANCY AND BREASTFEEDING – unless labelled as hepatotoxic-pyrrolizidine alkaloid-free – possibly teratogenic, excreted in breast milk.

Contraindications and precautions: Ensure commercial products labelled as free from hepatotoxic-pyrrolizidine alkaloids. Do not use on broken skin. Avoid with liver disease, obstetric cholestasis. Avoid in those sensitive to plants in the Asteraceae/Compositae family – chrysanthemums, marigolds, daisies. Do not confuse with golden ragwort, Tansy.

Adverse effects: Hepatotoxic pyrrolizidine is toxic to the liver, lungs; carcinogenic, mutagenic, allergic reactions.

Interactions: Significant risk of interaction with carbamazepine, phenobarbital, phenytoin, rifampicin. Herbs containing hepatotoxic-pyrrolizidine alkaloids: boneset, borage, butterbur, coltsfoot, comfrey, forget-me-not, hemp agrimony, hound's tongue. Senecio species plants: dusty miller, golden ragwort, groundsel. Also echinacea, garlic, liquorice, St John's wort, schisandra.

RASPBERRY KETONE

4-(4-Hydroxyphenyl)butan-2-one Aromatic substance found in red raspberries, cranberries, blackberries, kiwifruit, rhubarb.

Indications: Orally – for weight loss. Topically – for alopecia.

Safety in pregnancy: Commercial products often combined with caffeine to increase metabolism – advise normal cautions applicable to caffeine consumption in pregnancy. Caution: insufficient information on safety of raspberry ketone in isolation in pregnancy. Postnatally – advise caution.

Contraindications and precautions: Avoid in diabetics – may cause hypoglycaemia.

Adverse effects: Palpitations and jitteriness, possibly due to chemical similarity to stimulant, synephrine. Also hypertension, nausea.

Interactions: Therapeutic oral doses, prolonged, excessive or inappropriate use may interact with anticoagulants and antiplatelet drugs: heparin, warfarin, aspirin, diclofenac, ibuprofen, enoxaparin. Also antidiabetic medication, stimulant drugs: amphetamine, caffeine and others. Herbs: bitter melon, bitter orange, caffeine, chromium, coffee, cola nut, devil's claw, ephedra, fenugreek, garlic, horse chestnut, Panax ginseng, psyllium, Siberian ginseng.

RASPBERRY LEAF

Rubus idaeus Herbal remedy, also called Red raspberry leaf.

Indications: Orally – popularly used to prepare for labour – fragarine content thought to tone smooth muscle, aid cervical ripening, shorten duration of pregnancy and first stage of labour. Also prescribed by medical herbalists to prevent/treat threatened miscarriage, for pregnancy sickness, dysmenorrhoea, menorrhagia, gastrointestinal disorders, respiratory infections, cardiovascular disease, hypertension, diabetes mellitus, vitamin deficiencies, diarrhoea, as a diuretic, to enhance immune system, stimulate bile production, purify blood. Topically – for skin rashes and inflammation.

Safety in pregnancy: Appears safe in amounts commonly used in foods. Avoid in first and second trimesters unless prescribed by a qualified medical herbalist. If self-administered in third trimester, start with one cup of tea/one commercially prepared tablet daily for one week, increase gradually to two, then three a day over a three-week period; do not exceed three tablets daily unless professionally prescribed. Tea can be drunk in labour until well established – excessive consumption may cause hypertonic uterine action. Can be taken in early postnatal period to aid involution: advise women to withdraw slowly over two to three weeks to avoid myometrial relaxation (negative feedback). Intended as a *partus preparator* (preparation for birth) – should NOT be advised to start labour.

Contraindications and precautions: Do not use before 30 weeks unless under the supervision of a qualified medical herbalist. If taking as birth preparation in third trimester, reduce if Braxton Hicks contractions become uncomfortable or excessive. Do not exceed suggested doses – excessive amounts may delay, rather than facilitate, labour onset and duration of first stage. Do not delay starting raspberry leaf until term to avoid induction of labour – may cause uterine hypertonia, fetal distress. Do not take in conjunction with oxytocic drugs to stimulate contractions. Do not use concomitantly with Clary sage, Evening primrose oil, Castor oil, Black cohosh, Blue cohosh and other herbs taken to aid labour onset. Question women about self-administration of herbal remedies to initiate labour and record in notes. Obstetric contraindications: scar on uterus from previous Caesarean or other uterine surgery, planned Caesarean section, abnormal fetal presentation or lie, multiple pregnancy, low-lying placenta, placenta praevia, antepartum haemorrhage, vaginal spotting, history of preterm labour in previous pregnancy or threatened preterm labour in this pregnancy, history of previous precipitate labour, intrauterine growth retardation, other fetal compromise. Medical conditions (particularly smooth muscle systems) – epilepsy, major cardiovascular or cardiac conditions, pre-existing or gestational hypertension, major varicosities, thrombophlebitis, deep vein thrombosis, irritable bowel syndrome, Crohn's disease, diverticulitis, other gastrointestinal conditions, with anticoagulants/other drugs with anticoagulant action, history of coagulation disorder, hormone-sensitive conditions – ovarian, uterine and cervical cancer, fibroids, endometriosis, medication-controlled diabetes mellitus. Avoid if allergic to raspberries or strawberries. Do not confuse with raspberry fruit, Raspberry ketone.

Adverse effects: Oestrogenic effects may cause miscarriage, preterm, precipitate labour, hypertonic uterine action. Vasoconstrictive effects may cause hypertension. Also allergic reactions; diarrhoea, increased micturition.

Interactions: Therapeutic oral doses, prolonged, excessive or inappropriate use may interact with drugs and herbs with oxytocic action, vasoconstrictive drugs. Also anticoagulants and antiplatelet drugs: heparin, warfarin, aspirin, diclofenac, ibuprofen, enoxaparin. Antidiabetic medication, insulin. High iron content may interfere with absorption of zinc unless taken with food. Anticoagulant herbs: angelica, clove, fenugreek, feverfew, garlic, ginger, ginkgo, Panax ginseng, poplar, red clover, turmeric. Oestrogenic herbs: black cohosh, blue cohosh, dong quai, evening primrose, fennel, fenugreek, ginkgo, ginseng, liquorice, red clover, vitex agnus castus.

RED CLOVER
Trifolium pratense Herbal remedy.

Indications: Orally – for menopausal, postmenopausal symptoms, hot flushes, mastalgia, premenstrual syndrome. Also for osteoporosis, cancer prevention, indigestion, hypercholesterolaemia, whooping cough, asthma, bronchitis, sexually transmitted diseases. Topically – for dermatitis, burns, sore eyes, eczema and psoriasis.

Safety in pregnancy: Appears safe in amounts commonly found in foods. AVOID THERAPEUTIC ORAL DOSES IN PREGNANCY – contains phytoestrogens, structurally similar to oestradiol: oestrogenic effects may cause miscarriage. Safety of topical use – no information found.

Contraindications and precautions: Personal or family history of oestrogen-dependent conditions – breast, ovarian and uterine cancer, endometriosis, fibroids.

Adverse effects: Orally – weight gain, breast tenderness, skin irritation, headache, nausea.

Interactions: Therapeutic oral doses, prolonged, excessive or inappropriate use may interact with or potentiate oestrogens, hormone replacement therapy, tamoxifen, contraceptive Pill. Also possible interaction with anticoagulants, antiplatelet drugs, non-steroidal anti-inflammatories: heparin, warfarin, aspirin, diclofenac, ibuprofen, enoxaparin. Also amitriptyline, ondansetron, propranolol, theophylline, verapamil, diazepam. Herbs: alfalfa, angelica, clove, flaxseed, garlic, ginger, ginkgo, hops, horse chestnut, kudzu, liquorice, Panax ginseng, soy, turmeric. Oestrogenic herbs: black cohosh, blue cohosh, dong quai, evening primrose, fennel, fenugreek, raspberry leaf, vitex agnus castus.

RED RASPBERRY LEAF *see* Raspberry leaf

RESCUE REMEDY

Commercial preparation Combining extracts of five of the 38 Bach Flower remedies: cherry plum, clematis, impatiens, rock rose, Star of Bethlehem.

Indications: Stress, anxiety, panic, hysteria.

Safety in pregnancy: Orally and topically – appears safe in pregnancy, labour, postnatally, for babies, children. Available in liquid, cream, lozenge forms.

Contraindications and precautions: Flower extracts preserved in aqueous grape juice (alcohol) – avoid with obstetric cholestasis and other liver compromise, alcohol dependency. Aims to treat emotional issues – avoid with severe mental health problems, especially if on medication. Not to be used as a replacement for counselling or formal mental health consultation.

Adverse effects: Nausea and vomiting especially if taken with drugs (below) or alcohol. Prolonged inappropriate use of Rescue Remedy and other Bach Flower Remedies may mask worsening mental health problem.

Interactions: Therapeutic oral doses, prolonged, excessive or inappropriate use may interact with medication for drug dependency, alcohol, metronidazole.

RHUBARB

Rheum officinale, Rheum palmatum Herbal remedy, also known as Chinese rhubarb, Da huang.

Indications: Orally – for constipation, diarrhoea, haemorrhoids, heartburn, gastrointestinal bleeding. Also for pregnancy-induced hypertension, menopausal symptoms, dysmenorrhoea, gonorrhoea, hypercholesterolaemia, weight loss, pancreatitis, chronic kidney disease, sepsis, pesticide poisoning, certain cancers, non-alcoholic fatty liver disease. Topically – for cold sores. Rectally – for acute pancreatitis.

Safety in pregnancy: Stem safe in amounts commonly used in foods. AVOID THERAPEUTIC ORAL, RECTAL USE IN PREGNANCY. Possibly safe in therapeutic doses in postnatal period. Topically – no information available on safety – caution. Avoid leaf completely – poisonous.

Contraindications and precautions: Avoid with diarrhoea, intestinal obstruction, appendicitis, Crohn's disease, colitis, irritable bowel syndrome. Avoid with kidney disease, renal calculi – oxalic acid increases risk of stone formation. Avoid with liver disease – tannin may increase risk of hepatic toxicity. Do not confuse with Ma huang.

Adverse effects: Orally – therapeutic doses may cause cramping gastrointestinal discomfort, watery diarrhoea, nausea, vomiting, abdominal pain, uterine contractions, skin rash, allergic reactions leading to anaphylaxis, discoloured urine. Long-term use may lead to electrolyte loss, bone deterioration, proteinuria, haematuria, dehydration, inhibition of gastric motility, cardiac arrhythmias, muscular weakness, oedema, hepatotoxicity. Leaf is poisonous – oxalic acid may cause abdominal pain, burning of mouth and throat, diarrhoea, nausea, vomiting, seizures, death.

Interactions: Therapeutic oral doses, prolonged, excessive or inappropriate use may interact with warfarin, corticosteroids, diuretics, diclofenac, ibuprofen, naproxen, carbamazepine, nitrofurantoin, tamoxifen, laxatives, calcium, iron, zinc. Herbs: alder buckthorn, aloe, black hellebore, butternut bark, Canadian hemp root, comfrey, digitalis leaf, European buckthorn, figwort, greater bindweed, hedge mustard, horsetail, lily of the valley, liquorice, motherwort, oleander leaf, pennyroyal oil, red yeast, senna, yellow dock.

RHUS TOXICODENDRON
Homeopathic remedy from poison ivy, also known as Rhus tox.

Obstetric indications: For inflammation, joint and ligament pain, abdominal pain in pregnancy, afterpains, backache.

Key features: Aching, sore, bruised, tearing, stich-like ligamentous pain; improves with gentle movement, often followed by tiredness, return of pain. Uncomfortable in any position, restless, constantly moving around. Characteristically, feels better for sweating but then feels chilled. Dislikes any cold – food, drink, washing or swimming in cold water, cold wet weather.

Emotional symptoms: Restless – due to pain or nervousness; tosses and turns in bed, especially after midnight. Anxious, confused; mild but constant depression, often bursting into tears for no reason.

Better for: Changing position; fresh air; movement; sweating; warmth; hot drinks.

Worse for: Changing cloudy, cold, wet or damp weather, especially autumn; cold drinks; draughts; on beginning to move; lying down.

Safety: Do not confuse with poison ivy, herbal remedy. Do not use if there are any medical or obstetric complications. Not to be used as a replacement for standard medical care. Do not use with aromatherapy essential oils, topically or by inhalation, or with antacids, decongestants, laxatives or cough lozenges – inactivates the remedy. Do not take with food or drink. Do not take prophylactically – may lead to reverse proving. Should not be used by women who do not fit the symptom picture to avoid reverse proving. Caution: differentiate between Rhus tox (for ligament damage) and Ruta graveolens (for tendon pain) to avoid reverse proving. To be handled by the intended recipient only.

ROSE
Rosa centifolia Herbal remedy.

Indications: Topically – essential oil in aromatherapy used for relaxation, stress relief, anxiety, mild depression, insomnia, fatigue, constipation, nausea, pain relief, skin conditions, to prevent infection, stimulate immune system, as an aphrodisiac and for loss of libido.

Safety in pregnancy: AVOID TOPICAL OR INHALATIONAL USE OF ESSENTIAL OIL UNTIL LATE PREGNANCY – contains oestrogenic, emmenagoguic constituents, may cause miscarriage, preterm labour. Appears safe for topical and inhalational use from around 34 weeks' gestation in doses up to 1.5% in pregnancy and 2% in labour and postnatally.

Contraindications and precautions: Essential oil, topically or by inhalation – avoid with hay fever and asthma triggered by flower pollen – may have psychosomatic effect. Avoid if allergic to roses. Do not inhale directly from bottle or use in poorly ventilated room – contains phenols that irritate respiratory tract. Avoid rose absolute, sometimes used in aromatherapy although more often in perfumery – too concentrated for pregnancy use. Purchase from a reputable supplier – inexpensive brands may be adulterated with other natural or synthetic oils. Do not ingest. Do not use neat on skin or directly in a birthing pool. Do not use concomitantly with oxytocic drugs to expedite labour. Use a diffuser for a maximum of 15–20 minutes in any hour; do not vaporize in the second stage of labour to avoid neonatal exposure; do not diffuse near neonates, elderly or ill people. Do not diffuse in public areas or use excessive amounts which spread to public areas of maternity unit, to avoid excessive exposure of the woman, baby, visitors and staff to potential adverse effects. Caution with retained products of conception, emmenagoguic effect may precipitate haemorrhage. Do not apply directly to breasts in postnatal period, or wash with water before the baby starts feeding to avoid adverse neonatal effects from ingestion. Discontinue use if any allergic reactions occur to avoid accumulative reaction to specific chemicals – may lead to anaphylactic shock in severe cases. Do not use with or store near homeopathic remedies. Store in a refrigerator to avoid rapid oxidation. See also Rosehip.

Adverse effects: Topically – skin irritation, redness, burning, photosensitivity. By inhalation – nasal, throat inflammation, irritation, coughing. Prolonged inhalation, especially by infants and young children, may cause pneumonitis or pneumonia. Ingestion – nausea, vomiting, diarrhoea, dyspnoea, convulsions, coma.

Interactions: None documented, but in view of its mild oxytocic effect, advise caution with oxytocic drugs. Caution with oestrogenic herbs: black cohosh, blue cohosh, dong quai, evening primrose, fennel, fenugreek, ginkgo, ginseng, liquorice, raspberry leaf, red clover, vitex agnus castus.

ROSE GERANIUM *see* Geranium

ROSE OF SHARON *see* Hibiscus

ROSEHIP
Rosa canina, Rosa lutetiana Herbal remedy.

Indications: Orally – for common cold, influenza, vitamin C deficiency, gastrointestinal conditions, gallstones, urinary tract disorders, oedema, gout, arthritis, sciatica, diabetes mellitus, weight loss, increasing peripheral circulation. Topically – to prevent striae gravidarum.

Safety in pregnancy: Appears safe in amounts commonly used in foods or orally when prescribed by a qualified medical herbalist.

Contraindications and precautions: Diabetes mellitus, gout, renal calculi, thromboembolic conditions, glucose 6 phosphate dehydrogenase (G6PD), iron deficiency anaemia, thalassaemia, sickle cell disease. Excessive vitamin C content may interfere with results of laboratory tests for calcium, sodium, bilirubin, creatinine, glucose, occult blood, uric acid.

Adverse effects: Orally – nausea, vomiting, heartburn, abdominal cramps, gastrointestinal obstruction, diarrhoea; headache, insomnia, frequency of micturition, disturbances in urates, oxalate, cysteine. Adverse effects appear dose dependent; excessive amounts may cause deep vein thrombosis, kidney stones. Topically – contact dermatitis from rosehip dust.

Interactions: Therapeutic oral doses, prolonged, excessive or inappropriate use may interact with anticoagulants and antiplatelet drugs: heparin, warfarin, aspirin, diclofenac, ibuprofen, enoxaparin. Also aluminium, oestrogens, certain antipsychotic medication, lithium, iron, vitamin C. Anticoagulant herbs: angelica, clove, fenugreek, feverfew, garlic, ginger, ginkgo, Panax ginseng, poplar, red clover, turmeric.

ROSELLE *see* Hibiscus

ROSEMARY
Rosmarinus officinalis Herbal medicine.

Indications: Orally – to induce miscarriage, increase menstrual flow, for heartburn, flatulence, loss of appetite, cough, headache, opioid withdrawal, sun protection. Also to improve concentration and memory, increase energy levels, relieve stress, for depression, insomnia, hypertension or hypotension, hepatobiliary complaints. Topically and by inhalation, essential oil in aromatherapy – for mental alertness, as an analgesic, expectorant, bronchodilator, anti-inflammatory. Also topically for hair and scalp conditions, toothache; eczema, sciatica, wound healing; as an insect repellent.

Safety in pregnancy: Appears safe in amounts commonly used in foods. AVOID THERAPEUTIC AMOUNTS ORALLY, TOPICALLY OR BY INHALATION IN PREGNANCY, LABOUR OR BREASTFEEDING – may have abortifacient effects and increase oestrogen metabolism, leading to miscarriage, preterm labour. Camphor ketone is hepatotoxic, abortifacient.

Contraindications and precautions: Avoid excessive amounts in cooking; do not consume rosemary tea. Avoid with known aspirin allergy, epilepsy, coagulation and haemorrhagic disorders.

Adverse effects: Orally – excessive ingestion of herbal remedy, including tea, or undiluted essential oil may cause uterine bleeding, vomiting, kidney irritation, pulmonary oedema, coma, death. Convulsions may occur in rosemary containing high levels of camphor. Topically – photosensitivity, dermatitis. Repeated inhalation of oil may cause asthma.

Interactions: Therapeutic oral doses, prolonged, excessive or inappropriate oral or topical use or excessive inhalation may interact with anticoagulants and antiplatelet drugs: heparin, warfarin, aspirin, diclofenac, ibuprofen, enoxaparin. Also theophylline, propranolol, ondansetron, diazepam, iron supplements. Herbs: angelica, clove, garlic, ginger, ginkgo, meadowsweet, Panax ginseng, poplar, red clover, turmeric, willow bark.

ROYAL JELLY
Animal product from bee saliva.

Indications: Orally – for premenstrual syndrome, infertility, menopausal symptoms. Also for asthma, hay fever, to stimulate immune system, hepatitis, diabetes mellitus, insomnia, stomach ulcers, kidney disease, bone fractures, skin disorders, hyperlipidaemia. Topically – as a skin tonic and to stimulate hair growth.

Safety in pregnancy: Appears safe when used orally or topically, appropriately, short-term.

Contraindications and precautions: Avoid with asthma, coagulation or haemorrhagic disorders, hypotension, known allergy to bee pollen or genetic tendency to allergic reactions.

Adverse effects: Orally – hypersensitivity allergic reactions, status asthmaticus in known asthmatics. Topically, skin irritation, contact dermatitis.

Interactions: Therapeutic oral doses, prolonged, excessive or inappropriate use may interact with anticoagulants and antiplatelet drugs: heparin, warfarin, aspirin, diclofenac, ibuprofen, enoxaparin. Also antihypertensives. Herbs: angelica, cat's claw, clove, coenzyme Q10, fenugreek, feverfew, garlic, ginger, ginkgo, Panax ginseng, red clover, stinging nettle, turmeric, willow bark.

RUE
Ruta graveolens Herbal remedy; see also Ruta graveolens, homeopathic remedy.

Indications: Orally – for menstrual disorders, as abortifacient, uterine stimulant, for contraception. Also for loss of appetite, heartburn, circulatory disorders, palpitations, nervousness, hysteria, hepatitis, diarrhoea, headaches, respiratory conditions, as a diuretic, antibacterial, antifungal, haemostatic. Topically – for arthritis, sprains and bone injuries, skin inflammation, earache, toothache, headache, as an insect repellent.

Safety in pregnancy: AVOID ORAL USE IN PREGNANCY AND LABOUR – uterine stimulant and abortifacient.

Contraindications and precautions: Gastrointestinal, renal, hepatic conditions. Do not confuse with homeopathic Ruta graveolens.

Adverse effects: Orally, fresh leaves – renal and kidney damage, gastrointestinal disorders, sleep disturbance, bradycardia, death. Dried leaves have milder effects. Topically – contact dermatitis, photosensitivity. Oil – ingestion can cause severe stomach pain, vomiting, exhaustion, confusion, convulsions.

Interactions: Therapeutic oral doses, prolonged, excessive or inappropriate use may interact with photosensitizing drugs, for example chlorpromazine. Photosensitizing herbs: angelica, aniseed, bergamot, ginkgo, St John's wort.

RUTA GRAVEOLENS
Ruta graveolens Homeopathic remedy from rue.

Obstetric indications: Backache, sciatica in pregnancy, strains, sprains, tendon injury; bruised bones; headache, due to eyestrain.

Key features: Muscle and tendon strain due to over-exertion or injury; painful, bruised, stiff with weakness; lameness following injury; lower backache; injury to bones with sensation of aching and bruising; eyes – red, hot. First aid remedy for strains and sprains; also available as topical homeopathic cream.

Emotional symptoms: Restlessness; anxiety; quarrelsome; fear of death.

Better for: Movement; lying on back; rubbing affected area.

Worse for: Cold; during wet weather; lying down; overexertion; rest; night.

Safety: Do not use if there are any medical or obstetric complications. Not to be used as a replacement for standard medical care. Do not use with aromatherapy essential oils, topically or by inhalation, or with antacids, decongestants, laxatives or cough lozenges – inactivates the remedy. Do not take with food or drink. Do not take prophylactically – may lead to reverse proving. Should not be used by women who do not fit the symptom picture to avoid reverse proving. Do not confuse with Rue (*Ruta graveolens*), herbal remedy. Caution: differentiate between Ruta graveolens (for tendon pain) and Rhus toxicodendron (ligament damage) to avoid reverse proving. To be handled by the intended recipient only.

SABJA *see* Basil

SAGE
Salvia officinalis Herbal remedy.

Indications: Orally – for dysmenorrhoea, galactorrhoea, menopausal hot flushes. Also for loss of appetite, flatulence, bloating, heartburn, diarrhoea; excessive perspiration or saliva, depression, diabetes mellitus, post-surgical pain. Topically, essential oil in aromatherapy – for genital herpes, menopausal symptoms, laryngitis, tonsillitis, gingivitis, inflammation of nasal mucosa and to prevent sunburn. By inhalation – for asthma, to improve memory and cognitive function.

Safety in pregnancy: Avoid excessive consumption in food in pregnancy. AVOID THERAPEUTIC ORAL DOSES AND TOPICAL OR INHALATIONAL USE OF ESSENTIAL OIL IN PRECONCEPTION, ANTENATAL, INTRAPARTUM AND POSTNATAL PERIODS – thujone content may have strong emmenagoguic and abortifacient effects. Avoid oral use and topical or inhalational use of essential oil in postnatal period: may trigger postpartum haemorrhage, especially with retained products of conception; may reduce milk supply.

Contraindications and precautions: Diabetes mellitus, hypertension, hypotension, epilepsy, oestrogen-dependent conditions. Do not confuse with Clary sage.

Adverse effects: Orally – nausea, vomiting, abdominal pain, diarrhoea, dizziness, agitation. In high doses, can cause convulsions due to neurotoxic thujone, camphor, cineol; camphor can also cause hepatotoxicity. Topically – contact dermatitis, burning. Inhalation – wheezing and respiratory impairment.

Interactions: Therapeutic oral doses, prolonged, excessive or inappropriate use may interact with oestrogens, anticonvulsants, cimetidine, antidiabetic medication, antihypertensives, diclofenac, anticholinergic drugs, acetylcholinesterase inhibitors, benzodiazepines, central nervous system depressants, diazepam, fluoxetine, ondansetron, tramadol. Herbs: California poppy, catnip, cat's claw, coenzyme Q10, devil's claw, fenugreek, garlic, hops, horse chestnut seed, Jamaican dogwood, kava, Panax ginseng, psyllium, St John's wort, Siberian ginseng, skullcap, stinging nettle, valerian.

ST JOHN'S WORT

Hypericum perforatum Herbal remedy, also known as Hypericum.

Indications: Orally – for mild to moderate depression, mood disturbance, polycystic ovary syndrome, menopausal symptoms. Also for attention deficit-hyperactivity disorder, phobias, obsessive-compulsive disorder, seasonal affective disorder, smoking cessation, chronic fatigue syndrome, insomnia, irritable bowel syndrome. Topically – bruises, lacerations, wound healing, tooth extraction, psoriasis, haemorrhoids, cold sores, genital herpes.

Safety in pregnancy: AVOID ORAL USE IN PREGNANCY – some authorities believe it may be teratogenic, although evidence is inconclusive. AVOID IN BREASTFEEDING – neonates of women who take it in pregnancy or whilst breastfeeding may have greater risk of colic, lethargy, drowsiness.

Contraindications and precautions: Do not substitute prescribed antidepressants with St John's wort – mechanism of action similar to selective serotonin reuptake inhibitors (SSRIs): withdrawal should be gradual/monitored to avoid symptoms similar to SSRI withdrawal. Do not take antidepressant medication and St John's wort concomitantly. Avoid with infertility. Do not confuse with homeopathic Hypericum.

Adverse effects: Insomnia, vivid dreams, restlessness, anxiety, panic attacks, irritability, agitation, dizziness, headache, skin rashes, hypoglycaemia, hypertension, photosensitivity. Rarely, serious effects similar to those with SSRIs, namely SSRI syndrome, usually due to rapid withdrawal: suicidal thoughts and mania. May elevate thyroid-stimulating hormone levels. Abnormal menstrual bleeding when taken concomitantly with contraceptive Pill.

Interactions: Therapeutic oral doses, prolonged, excessive or inappropriate use may interact with antidepressants, notably SSRIs, sertraline, tricyclics; contraceptive Pill; antirejection drugs, for example cyclosporine for transplant patients; verapamil, fentanyl, glucocorticoids, digoxin, certain cancer drugs, ketamine, some anticonvulsants, antiretroviral drugs, pentazocine, phenobarbital, phenytoin, theophylline, tryptophan, warfarin, iron supplements, many more drugs. Serotonergic herbs: Hawaiian baby woodrose, L-tryptophan. Also red yeast.

SARSAPARILLA

Smilax febrifuga Herbal remedy.

Indications: Orally – for skin diseases, rheumatoid arthritis, renal disease, athletic performance, as a diuretic, for leprosy, syphilis.

Safety in pregnancy: Appears safe in amounts commonly used in foods or in moderate oral therapeutic doses.

Contraindications and precautions: Asthma, kidney disease.

Adverse effects: Asthma from inhalation of root dust.

Interactions: Therapeutic oral doses, prolonged, excessive or inappropriate use may interact with digoxin, lithium. Herbs: black hellebore, Canadian hemp root, digitalis leaf, figwort, lily of the valley, motherwort.

SASSAFRAS

Sassafras albidum, Sassafras officinale Herbal remedy.

Indications: Orally – for urinary tract disorders, mucous membrane inflammation, bronchitis, hypertension, arthritis, skin problems, kidney disorders, cancers, as a general tonic. Topically – for skin conditions, eye inflammation, sprains, oedema, insect bites, stings, as an antiseptic.

Safety in pregnancy: AVOID THERAPEUTIC ORAL OR TOPICAL DOSES IN PREGNANCY – abortifacient, may be carcinogenic, hepatotoxic. Advise caution: insufficient information on safety when breastfeeding.

Contraindications and precautions: Urinary tract conditions – may aggravate irritation.

Adverse effects: Orally – miscarriage, diaphoresis, hot flushes, hallucinations, vomiting, dilated pupils, hypertension, tachycardia, collapse, carcinoma, death. Topically – contact dermatitis.

Interactions: Therapeutic oral doses, prolonged, excessive or inappropriate use may interact with central nervous system depressants and sedatives. Sedative herbs: calamus, California poppy, catnip, hops, Jamaican dogwood, kava, St John's wort, skullcap, valerian. Safrole-containing herbs: basil, camphor, cinnamon, nutmeg.

SATAVAR *see* Shatavari

SAW PALMETTO

Serenoa repens Herbal remedy.

Indications: Orally – to increase breast size, for chronic pelvic pain syndrome, to improve libido, as an aphrodisiac. Most commonly for benign prostatic hyperplasia, other prostate problems. Also for common cold, coughs, sore throat, chronic bronchitis, migraine, cancer; as a diuretic and sedative. Topically – for alopecia, hirsutism. Vaginally, as uterine and vaginal tonic.

Safety in pregnancy: AVOID ORAL AND INTRAVAGINAL USE IN PREGNANCY – oestrogenic effects.

Contraindications and precautions: Avoid with haemorrhagic and coagulation disorders – may prolong bleeding time. May interfere with results of liver function tests. Discontinue use prior to surgery.

Adverse effects: Orally – dizziness, headache, nausea, vomiting, constipation, diarrhoea, loss of libido, ejaculation disorders, postural hypotension. May have anticoagulant and hepatotoxic effects.

Interactions: Therapeutic oral doses, prolonged, excessive or inappropriate use may interact with anticoagulants and antiplatelet drugs: heparin, warfarin, aspirin, diclofenac, ibuprofen, enoxaparin. Also contraceptive Pill, oestrogens. Anticoagulant herbs: angelica, clove, fenugreek, feverfew, garlic, ginger, ginkgo, Panax ginseng, poplar, red clover, turmeric. Oestrogenic herbs: black cohosh, blue cohosh, dong quai, evening primrose, fennel, liquorice, raspberry leaf, red clover, vitex agnus castus. May interfere with tests for clotting times and liver function.

SCHISANDRA
Schisandra chinensis Herbal remedy.

Indications: Orally – for stress reduction, motion sickness, premenstrual syndrome. Also as performance enhancer, to improve vision, normalize blood sugar and blood pressure, reduce cholesterol, for liver protection, postoperative recovery, to prevent premature ageing, for cough, asthma, insomnia, diarrhoea, impotence, depression, irritability, as an immunostimulant.

Safety in pregnancy: Fruit appears safe enough in amounts used in cooking. AVOID THERAPEUTIC ORAL DOSES IN PREGNANCY – may be uterine stimulant, potentially causing miscarriage, preterm labour.

Contraindications and precautions: Epilepsy – due to possible central nervous system stimulation. Caution with oesophageal reflux, heartburn.

Adverse effects: Heartburn, indigestion, decreased appetite, abdominal pain, allergic skin rashes, urticaria.

Interactions: Therapeutic oral doses, prolonged, excessive or inappropriate use may interact with anticoagulants and antiplatelet drugs: heparin, warfarin, aspirin, diclofenac, ibuprofen, enoxaparin. Anticoagulant herbs: angelica, clove, fenugreek, feverfew, garlic, ginger, ginkgo, Panax ginseng, poplar, red clover, turmeric.

SECALE
Secale cornutum Homeopathic remedy from ergot.

Obstetric indications: Labour contractions – weak, ineffectual, irregular or diminish totally; no expulsive activity; trembling when contractions cease; burning, spasmodic pain. Retained placenta with bearing-down sensation; retention of urine. Postpartum bleeding, afterpains, poor milk supply with stinging pain in breasts.

Key features: Restlessness; passive bleeding; strength drains quickly; dry, coarse skin; numbness, tingling; feels hot internally, but cold externally; offensive discharge; thin, dark brown lochia; trembling, twitching, spasms; reduced urine output; excessive thirst.

Emotional symptoms: Fearful; confusion, stupor; suspicion; doubts her sanity; shameless.

Better for: Uncovering, even though cold to touch; cold applications; cool fresh air.

Worse for: Warmth; being covered; great aversion to heat; minimal movement.

Safety: Controversy regarding homeopathic Secale for retained placenta, to antidote effects of oxytocic medication and control intrapartum bleeding. Do not use if there are any medical or obstetric complications. Not to be used as a replacement for standard medical care. Do not use in conjunction with standard oxytocics for the third stage of labour unless under the supervision of a qualified homeopath. Do not use with aromatherapy essential oils, topically or by inhalation, or with antacids, decongestants, laxatives or cough lozenges – inactivates the remedy. Do not take with food or drink. Do not take prophylactically – may lead to reverse proving. Should not be used by women who do not fit the symptom picture to avoid reverse proving. To be handled by the intended recipient only. Do not confuse with Ergot, herbal remedy.

SENNA

Senna alexandrina, Cassia acutifolia Herbal remedy.

Indications: Orally – for constipation, irritable bowel syndrome, haemorrhoids, anorectal surgery, anal fissures, weight loss.

Safety in pregnancy: Orally – appears safe in small doses, short-term. No apparent adverse effects on neonatal bowel movements if taken when breastfeeding.

Contraindications and precautions: Avoid with a history of threatened or repeated miscarriages; do not use as enematic preparation prior to labour – too purgative. Avoid with dehydration, diarrhoea, Crohn's disease, ulcerative colitis, appendicitis, stomach inflammation, anal prolapse, haemorrhoids, undiagnosed abdominal pain. May interfere with tests for electrolyte imbalance.

Adverse effects: Orally – abdominal pain, bloating, flatulence, nausea, bowel urgency, diarrhoea, asthma, allergy symptoms. Excessive use – depletion of potassium, other electrolytes, cardiovascular disorders, muscular weakness, liver damage, coma, neuropathy.

Interactions: Therapeutic oral doses, prolonged, excessive or inappropriate use may interact with contraceptive Pill, oestrogens, diuretics. Also anticoagulants: heparin, warfarin, aspirin. Herbs: horsetail, liquorice; stimulant herbs including aloe vera, black root, buckthorn, butternut bark, greater bindweed, rhubarb, senna, yellow dock.

SEPIA

Sepia officinalis Homeopathic remedy from cuttlefish ink.

Obstetric indications: Backache, carpal tunnel syndrome, constipation, faintness, insomnia, nausea worse after eating. Labour contractions severe, sharp, clutching, stitching, weak, ineffective; extend from cervix up into back or umbilicus; shudders during contractions. Also for premenstrual and menopausal symptoms, uterine prolapse with bearing-down sensation.

Key features: Run down and burned out. Sagging, bearing-down sensation in uterus/anus; weakness; exhausted, faint; feels cold, even in warm environment; sallow complexion. Prone to ulcers, herpes; lack of muscle tone. Sagging, pendulous breasts. Craves vinegar, pickles; averse to fats and sex.

Emotional symptoms: Exhausted, run down, depressed; indifferent towards loved ones; detached, irritable, easily offended; resentful if left unattended but rejects sympathy; fears something dreadful about to happen; may be tearful when relating symptoms; verbalizes "had enough".

Better for: After eating; being covered up; warmth; exercise; pressure; crossing limbs; lying on right side.

Worse for: Early evening and at night; lying on left side; tiredness; touch; damp conditions.

Safety: Do not use if there are any medical or obstetric complications. Not to be used as a replacement for standard medical care. Do not use with aromatherapy essential oils, topically or by inhalation, or with antacids, decongestants, laxatives or cough lozenges – inactivates the remedy. Do not take with food or drink. Do not take prophylactically – may lead to reverse proving. Should not be used by women who do not fit the symptom picture to avoid reverse proving. To be handled by the intended recipient only.

SHATAVARI

Asparagus racemosus Herbal remedy, also known as Satavar.

Indications: Orally – for uterine bleeding, premenstrual syndrome, to promote fertility, stimulate lactation. Also for pain, heartburn, constipation, diarrhoea, anxiety, alcohol withdrawal, bronchitis, diabetes mellitus, as a diuretic, antispasmodic, aphrodisiac, immunostimulant.

Safety in pregnancy: Orally – safe in amounts commonly found in foods. AVOID THERAPEUTIC ORAL DOSES IN PREGNANCY unless under the supervision of a qualified Ayurvedic practitioner or medical herbalist. Appears safe to use in moderate doses for lactation.

Contraindications and precautions: Do not confuse with asparagus (*Asparagus officinale*).

Adverse effects: Allergic reactions – skin irritation, rash, redness, dyspnoea, tachycardia, dizziness, eye irritation; also hypoglycaemia.

Interactions: Therapeutic oral doses, prolonged, excessive or inappropriate use may interact with diuretics, antidiabetic medication, lithium. Herbs: aloe, bitter melon, cinnamon, fenugreek, ginger, ginseng, kudzu, marshmallow, milk thistle, schisandra.

SHEPHERD'S PURSE

Capsella bursa-pastoris Herbal remedy, also known as Lady's purse.

Indications: Orally – for headache, hypotension, premenstrual complaints, menorrhagia, dysmenorrhoea, haematuria, diarrhoea, cystitis. Topically – for nose bleeds, burns, skin injuries.

Safety in pregnancy: AVOID ORAL USE IN PREGNANCY – may cause uterine contractions, miscarriage, preterm labour. Topical use appears safe. Advise caution: insufficient information on safety when breastfeeding.

Contraindications and precautions: Kidney disease, thyroid disease.

Adverse effects: Theoretical risk of nitrate toxicity.

Interactions: Therapeutic oral doses, prolonged, excessive or inappropriate use may interact with sedatives, thyroid hormones. Sedative herbs: calamus, California poppy, catnip, hops, Jamaican dogwood, kava, St John's wort, skullcap, valerian.

SHIKOR MATI/SIKOR *see* Calabash chalk

SIBERIAN GINSENG

Eleutherococcus senticosus Herbal remedy, also known as Eleuthero.

Indications: Orally – for stress, chronic fatigue syndrome, influenza, chronic bronchitis, improving athletic performance, hangover symptoms, herpes simplex, insomnia, attention deficit-hyperactivity disorder, diabetes mellitus, pyelonephritis, hypertension, as a diuretic, appetite stimulant, immunostimulant.

Safety in pregnancy: Orally – appears relatively safe in pregnancy in small amounts but little information is available about safety – risk of adverse effects may outweigh potential benefits, mask obstetric complications – caution.

Contraindications and precautions: Avoid with haemorrhagic disorders, pre-existing or gestational diabetes, hormone-sensitive conditions – breast, uterine and ovarian cancer, endometriosis, fibroids; hypertension, mental health disorders. Commercial products may be adulterated with other herbal constituents. Do not confuse with Asian/Chinese/Korean red ginseng (*Panax ginseng*).

Adverse effects: Contact dermatitis, anxiety, irritability, hypertension, nausea, diarrhoea, breast tenderness, headache.

Interactions: Therapeutic oral doses, prolonged, excessive or inappropriate use may interact with alcohol, anticoagulants, antiplatelet drugs, diabetic medication;

pentazocine, theophylline, amitriptyline, diazepam, verapamil, oestradiol, immunosuppressants, lithium, cimetidine, ranitidine. Anticoagulant and antiplatelet herbs: angelica, clove, garlic, ginger, Panax ginseng, red clover, turmeric. Hypoglycaemic herbs: bitter melon, fenugreek, ginger, kudzu. Sedative herbs: California poppy, catnip, German chamomile, gotu kola, hops, Jamaican dogwood, kava, lemon balm, sage, St John's wort, sassafras, skullcap, valerian.

SILICA

Silicea terra Homeopathic remedy, tissue salt from flint (mineral), also known as Silicea.

Obstetric indications: Constipation, backache, common cold. Sore nipples with bleeding, breast abscess.

Key features: Easily exhausted; hardening of glandular tissue; extremely sensitive to cold; no energy or willpower; restless, gradual onset and resolution of symptoms, generally left sided; localized numbness, heaviness; sharp, cutting, sore pain.

Emotional symptoms: Weak, lacks stamina and confidence, absentminded, morbid dreams. Nervous, shy, sensitive, startles easily, cries when spoken to. Fear of failure and of pointed objects (needle phobia).

Better for: Warmth; wrapping the head; summer; wet or humid weather.

Worse for: Cold weather; loud noises; mental exertion; evening and night; lying on painful side.

Safety: Do not use if there are any medical or obstetric complications. Not to be used as a replacement for standard medical care. Do not use with aromatherapy essential oils, topically or by inhalation, or with antacids, decongestants, laxatives or cough lozenges – inactivates the remedy. Do not take with food or drink. Do not take prophylactically – may lead to reverse proving. Should not be used by women who do not fit the symptom picture to avoid reverse proving. To be handled by the intended recipient only.

SKULLCAP

Scutellaria lateriflora Herbal remedy, also known as American/Blue skullcap, Blue pimpernel.

Indications: Orally – for insomnia, anxiety, premenstrual disorders. Also for pyrexia, hyperlipidaemia, atherosclerosis, nervous tension, allergies, dermatitis, inflammation.

Safety in pregnancy: Orally – safe in pregnancy and breastfeeding under the supervision of a qualified medical herbalist; insufficient information on safety – advise caution with self-administration.

Contraindications and precautions: Do not confuse with Chinese skullcap (*Scutellaria baicalensis*). Commercial products may contain different types of skullcap or be adulterated with other herbs such as germander.

Adverse effects: Digestive disturbance, sedation, cognitive impairment; hepatotoxicity in large doses.

Interactions: Therapeutic oral doses, prolonged, excessive or inappropriate use may interact with sedatives, anaesthetics, morphine, fentanyl, benzodiazepines. Herbs: California poppy, catnip, hops, Jamaican dogwood, kava, St John's wort, valerian.

SLIPPERY ELM

Ulmus rubra Herbal remedy, also known as Indian elm.

Indications: Orally – for pregnancy sickness, to facilitate labour, as abortifacient, for diarrhoea, constipation, haemorrhoids, irritable bowel syndrome, cystitis. Also for cough, sore throat, colic, to prevent stomach and duodenal ulcers. Intracervically – as abortifacient. Topically – as a lubricant to ease childbirth, wounds, burns, cold sores, toothache.

Safety in pregnancy: Teas and supplements from inner bark appear safe enough. AVOID THERAPEUTIC ORAL AND INTRACERVICAL USE OF OUTER BARK IN PREGNANCY unless under the supervision of a qualified medical herbalist – may cause miscarriage.

Contraindications and precautions: Do not use if on any medication – may interfere with absorption. Commercially produced teas may not state which part of the bark has been used.

Adverse effects: Topically – skin irritation.

Interactions: Theoretical risk of inhibition of any medication taken orally – sticky mucilage content may impair absorption and reduce amount of circulating drug.

SNAKEWEED *see* Euphorbia

SPANISH THYME *see* Thyme

SPIKENARD

Nardostachys jatamansi Herbal remedy, also known as Jatamansi.

Indications: Topically and by inhalation, essential oil in aromatherapy – for muscular pain, headache, dysmenorrhoea, bacterial and fungal infections, constipation, to reduce inflammation. Orally in Ayurvedic medicine – for dysmenorrhoea, menopausal symptoms, to tone uterus, antibacterial, anti-inflammatory, laxative, to aid sleep, enhance memory, for relaxation.

Safety in pregnancy: AVOID ORAL THERAPEUTIC DOSES IN PREGNANCY unless under the supervision of a qualified Ayurvedic practitioner. Topically and by inhalation, essential oil – insufficient information available on safety in pregnancy and breastfeeding – advise caution.

Contraindications and precautions: Do not ingest essential oil. Do not use with any medical or obstetric condition. Do not diffuse for more than 15–20 minutes in one hour; do not diffuse in public areas of maternity unit or near neonates, elderly or ill people. Do not use neat or add to a birthing pool. Considered endangered species due to over-cultivation.

Adverse effects: Orally – nausea, vomiting, diarrhoea, abdominal pain and cramping, frequency of micturition. Topically – skin irritation, contact dermatitis, erythema, inflammation, allergic reactions.

Interactions: None documented.

SQUAW VINE
Mitchella repens Herbal remedy, also known as Partridge berry, Deerberry.

Indications: Orally – to facilitate and shorten duration of labour, improve lactation, for postnatal depression, to induce miscarriage; for amenorrhoea, menorrhagia, dysmenorrhoea, leucorrhoea. Also for anxiety, diarrhoea, oedema, fibrocystic breast disease, oliguria, insomnia, congestive heart failure, kidney failure, liver failure. Topically – for sore nipples.

Safety in pregnancy: AVOID THERAPEUTIC ORAL DOSES IN FIRST AND SECOND TRIMESTERS – emmenagoguic, may cause miscarriage. Appears safe to use from third trimester under the supervision of a qualified medical herbalist but advise against self-administration. Topically – appears safe for sore nipples, but advise application after feeding to reduce the impact of ingestion by the baby.

Contraindications and precautions: Avoid prolonged use. Avoid with obstetric cholestasis, pre-existing liver disease.

Adverse effects: Heartburn, mucous membrane irritation. Rarely – hepatotoxicity.

Interactions: Atropine, scopolamine, iron supplements, cardiac glycosides.

STAPHYSAGRIA
Delphinium staphysagria Homeopathic remedy from Larkspur/Delphinium.

Obstetric indications: Stinging, stitching, burning pain, cystitis; surgery with nerve involvement or incision going across natural lines of body; epidural anaesthesia. Sense of humiliation or violation from invasive medical procedures, for example vaginal examinations, catheterization, forceps delivery, episiotomy.

Key features: Raw, sore tissues with burning, stinging; burning after micturition; lacerated tissues; clenched teeth and jaw; violent itching. Headache with boring sensation, mainly forehead. Symptoms triggered by offensive comments; physically and emotionally hypersensitive.

Emotional symptoms: Tends to mask feelings; prefers solitude and to avoid confrontation; overly sensitive to criticism; tendency to overreact when emotions eventually explode.

Better for: Rest; warmth; good night's sleep.

Worse for: Sitting down; exertion; anger; indignation; sexual excesses; touch; pressure; dehydration.

Safety: Do not use if there are any medical or obstetric complications. Not to be used as a replacement for standard medical care. Do not use with aromatherapy essential oils, topically or by inhalation, or with antacids, decongestants, laxatives or cough lozenges – inactivates the remedy. Do not take with food or drink. Do not take prophylactically – may lead to reverse proving. Should not be used by women who do not fit the symptom picture to avoid reverse proving. To be handled by the intended recipient only. Do not confuse with Delphinium/Larkspur, herbal remedy – causes cardiac and respiratory failure.

STAR ANISE
Illicium verum Herbal remedy, also known as Chinese star anise.

Indications: Orally – to promote menstruation, aid labour, increase libido. Also for influenza, cough, bronchitis, gastrointestinal disturbance, flatulence, loss of appetite, infant colic. By inhalation – respiratory congestion.

Safety in pregnancy: Appears safe in amounts commonly used in foods. AVOID THERAPEUTIC ORAL DOSES AND INHALATION IN PREGNANCY – may be abortifacient, causing miscarriage, preterm labour.

Contraindications and precautions: Do not give to infants as tea – may cause gastrointestinal and neurological complications due to toxicity from contamination with Japanese star anise. Do not confuse with Japanese star anise (*Illicium anisatum*) – poisonous.

Adverse effects: None documented.

Interactions: None documented.

STINGING NETTLE
Urtica dioica, Urtica urens Herbal remedy.

Indications: Orally – for allergies, hay fever, eczema, uterine bleeding, nose bleeds, urinary tract infections, iron deficiency anaemia. Also for poor circulation, diabetes mellitus, as a diuretic. Topically – for musculoskeletal pain, dermatitis, oily hair, alopecia.

Safety in pregnancy: Safe for topical use and orally in amounts commonly used in foods. AVOID THERAPEUTIC ORAL USE IN PREGNANCY unless under the supervision of a qualified medical herbalist – excessive consumption may cause miscarriage, preterm labour.

Contraindications and precautions: Avoid with coagulation and haemorrhagic disorders, diabetes mellitus. Avoid with renal disease unless under the supervision of a qualified medical herbalist. Caution with hypotension, anaemias not due to iron deficiency.

Adverse effects: Orally – diarrhoea, constipation, headache, fatigue, allergic rhinitis. Topically – skin rash, itching, stinging, hypersensitivity to cold.

Interactions: Therapeutic oral doses, prolonged, excessive or inappropriate use may interact with anticoagulants and antiplatelet drugs: heparin, warfarin, aspirin, diclofenac, ibuprofen, enoxaparin. Also antidiabetic medication, antihypertensives, central nervous system depressants, lithium. Herbs: cat's claw, coenzyme Q10, devil's claw, fenugreek, fish oil, garlic, ginger, ginkgo, meadowsweet, Panax ginseng, Siberian ginseng, turmeric, willow bark.

STINKING NIGHTSHADE *see* Henbane

STINKING WILLIE *see* Ragwort

SWEET ALMOND
Prunus amygdalus var. dulcis, Amygdalus communis var. dulcis Herbal remedy.

Indications: Orally – as a laxative, for obesity, hypercholesterolaemia, cardiac disease, diabetes mellitus, various cancers. Topically – as an emollient for dry skin, to ease mucous membrane inflammation, for radiation dermatitis, as carrier oil in massage.

Safety in pregnancy: Orally – appears safe in amounts commonly used in foods. Topically – suitable for use as carrier oil for massage and aromatherapy.

Contraindications and precautions: Avoid oral or topical use if allergic specifically to almonds (rather than nuts in general). Diabetes mellitus – taken orally, may interfere with serum glucose. Do not confuse with Bitter almond.

Adverse effects: Excessive oral consumption of sweet almond milk, especially in children, or adults with pre-existing conditions, may increase risk of genitourinary problems and renal calculi due to oxalate content – ensure high water intake to dilute effects. Topically – skin irritation, erythema.

Interactions: Therapeutic oral doses, prolonged, excessive or inappropriate use may interact with antidiabetic medication. Hypoglycaemic herbs: devil's claw, fenugreek, Panax ginseng, Siberian ginseng.

SWEET FENNEL *see* Fennel

SWEET MARJORAM *see* Marjoram

TAMARIND
Tamarindus indica Herbal remedy.

Indications: Orally – for pregnancy sickness, constipation, digestive disorders, pyrexia, hepatobiliary disorders, common cold, worms. Topically – for fractures; as eye drops. Often used in Ayurvedic medicine.

Safety in pregnancy: Appears safe in amounts commonly found in foods. Insufficient information available on safety in pregnancy – advise cautious use of therapeutic oral doses unless under the supervision of a qualified Ayurvedic practitioner.

Contraindications and precautions: Avoid with diabetes mellitus, gestational diabetes.

Adverse effects: Inhalation of powder from dried seeds may cause cough, dyspnoea.

Interactions: Therapeutic oral doses, prolonged, excessive or inappropriate use may interact with antidiabetic medication, aspirin, ibuprofen. Hypoglycaemic herbs: devil's claw, fenugreek, guar gum, Panax ginseng, Siberian ginseng.

TANGERINE *see* Mandarin

TANSY
Tanacetum vulgare, *Chrysanthemum vulgare*, *Tanacetum boreale* Herbal remedy.

Indications: Orally – as abortifacient, for migraine headache, poor appetite, flatulence, gastrointestinal ulcers, hepatobiliary disease, common cold, as an antioxidant, antiseptic, antispasmodic, bactericide, emmenagogue, tonic. Topically – for scabies, pruritus, bruising, sores, sprains, swelling, inflammation, leucorrhoea, toothache, as an insect repellent.

Safety in pregnancy: Appears safe in amounts commonly used in foods. AVOID THERAPEUTIC ORAL AND TOPICAL USE IN PREGNANCY, LABOUR AND EARLY POSTNATAL PERIOD – thujone content is emmenagoguic, abortifacient, may cause miscarriage, preterm labour, hypertonic uterine contractions, excessive lochial discharges.

Contraindications and precautions: Avoid excessive consumption of tea in pregnancy. Avoid if allergy to plants in the Asteraceae/Compositae family – ragweed, chrysanthemums, marigolds, daisies. Do not confuse with Tansy ragwort. Do not confuse with chrysanthemum (*Chrysanthemum morifolium*) used for tea and in Chinese medicine – safe to drink in moderation.

Adverse effects: Thujone content possibly toxic when ingested, including consumption of tea, causing tachycardia, tachypnoea, gastroenteritis, dilated pupils, hepatotoxicity, nephrotoxicity, death. Topically – contact dermatitis, photosensitivity.

Interactions: Therapeutic oral doses, prolonged, excessive or inappropriate use may interact with alcohol. Thujone-containing herbs: oak moss, oriental arbor vitae, sage, thuga (cedar), tree moss, wormwood.

TANSY RAGWORT *see* Ragwort

TEA TREE
Melaleuca alternifolia Herbal remedy.

Indications: Topically, essential oil in aromatherapy – for skin conditions, thrush, vaginal infections, haemorrhoids, recurrent herpes labialis. Also for acne, athlete's foot, head lice; as local antiseptic for cuts, abrasions, burns, contact dermatitis, herpes simplex, dandruff, toothache, sore throat, ear infections. Used to prevent and treat hospital-acquired methicillin-resistant *Staphylococcus aureus*. By inhalation – for respiratory infections, common cold, sinusitis. In bath – for perineal healing following delivery.

Safety in pregnancy: Essential oil used in aromatherapy appears safe in doses up to 1.5% in pregnancy and 2% in postnatal period. AVOID IN LABOUR – relaxant effect on smooth muscle.

Contraindications and precautions: Essential oil, topically or by inhalation – do not use intravaginally for thrush and other infections during pregnancy or postnatal period – risk of mucous membrane irritation. Do not ingest – toxic. Caution when used in a bath for perineal healing – can cause irritation. Do not use undiluted on open wounds. Do not apply directly to breasts in postnatal period. Use a diffuser for a maximum of 15–20 minutes in any hour; do not diffuse near neonates, elderly or ill people. Do not diffuse near animals – toxic to cats and dogs. Do not diffuse in public areas or use excessive amounts which spread to public areas of maternity unit, to avoid excessive exposure of the woman, baby, visitors and staff to potential adverse effects. Discontinue use if any allergic reactions occur to avoid accumulative reaction to specific chemicals – may lead to anaphylactic shock in severe cases. Do not use with or store near homeopathic remedies. Store in a refrigerator to avoid rapid oxidation.

Adverse effects: Topically – skin and mucous membrane irritation, contact dermatitis, redness. Orally – confusion, disorientation, ataxia, coma, dyspnoea.

Interactions: None documented.

THUJA
Thuja occidentalis Herbal remedy, also known as Arborvitae, Cedar leaf.

Indications: Orally – for respiratory infections, bacterial skin infections, herpes simplex, osteoarthritis, as an expectorant, immunostimulant, diuretic, abortifacient. Topically, essential oil in aromatherapy – for joint and muscle pain, skin diseases, warts, as an insect repellent.

Safety in pregnancy: AVOID THERAPEUTIC ORAL AND TOPICAL USE IN PREGNANCY AND BREASTFEEDING – abortifacient, toxic – may cause miscarriage, preterm labour; may be toxic to neonates.

Contraindications and precautions: Avoid completely with epilepsy, autoimmune disease. Do not confuse with cedarwood (*Cedrus atlantica*) – although essential oil should also be avoided in pregnancy.

Adverse effects: None documented.

Interactions: Therapeutic oral doses, prolonged, excessive or inappropriate use may interact with anticonvulsants, immunostimulants, epilepsy medication.

THYME
Thymus vulgaris Herbal remedy, also known as Spanish thyme.

Indications: Orally – for bronchitis, sore throat, colic, flatulence, indigestion, diarrhoea, enuresis, skin disorders, to delay ageing process, as diuretic and urinary disinfectant. Topically – for laryngitis, tonsillitis, stomach upset, hair loss, halitosis, in mouthwashes.

Safety in pregnancy: Appears safe in amounts commonly used in foods. AVOID THERAPEUTIC ORAL, TOPICAL AND INHALATIONAL USE OF ESSENTIAL OIL IN PREGNANCY – uterine-stimulating effects may cause miscarriage, preterm labour.

Contraindications and precautions: Bleeding disorders, hormone-sensitive condition – breast, uterine and ovarian cancer, endometriosis, fibroids.

Adverse effects: Orally – gastrointestinal effects, headache, dizziness. Topically – skin irritation, contact dermatitis. Allergic reactions in those allergic to oregano.

Interactions: Therapeutic oral doses, prolonged, excessive or inappropriate use may interact with anticoagulants and antiplatelet drugs: heparin, warfarin, aspirin, diclofenac, ibuprofen, naproxen, enoxaparin. Also antihypertensives, oestrogens. Herbs: angelica, anise, asafoetida, capsicum, celery, chamomile, clove, fenugreek, feverfew, garlic, ginger, ginkgo, horse chestnut, liquorice, meadowsweet, Panax ginseng, passionflower, red clover, turmeric, willow bark.

TIGER BALM
Commercial over-the-counter herbal liniments, variously containing camphor, menthol, wintergreen, eucalyptus, spike lavender, salicylate, cassia cinnamon, capsicum, cajeput, clove.

Indications: Topically – for pain relief, mainly muscular and joint pain; headache, sinus congestion, cough, influenza symptoms, mosquito bites, to prevent/reduce stretch marks.

Safety in pregnancy: Safety information tends to distinguish between individual ingredients, citing eucalyptus as safe in pregnancy but urging caution with others; most information is based on evidence for safety of oral administration. Limited information on safety in pregnancy except generic advice to use sparingly. Breastfeeding – caution not to transfer ointment from maternal to neonatal skin: may be wise to avoid – inhalation of vapours may cause neonatal respiratory difficulties or allergy.

Contraindications and precautions: Do not take orally. Do not apply to burned, chapped or sore skin, or to open wounds. Do not use near eyes, in ears or groin. Do not cover skin to which applied. Do not use on babies, infants, young children. Do not use with other similar products or herbal remedies. Do not store near homeopathic remedies.

Adverse effects: Skin irritation, itching, stinging, burning; respiratory symptoms when used on chest for congestion. Allergic reactions, anaphylaxis.

Interactions: Theoretically, therapeutic dermal use, prolonged, excessive or inappropriate use may interact with anticoagulants, antihypertensives, antidiabetic medication, various other drugs – but evidence is based on oral administration of individual ingredients rather than topical use of commercially produced combination. No herbs identified.

TUKMARIA *see* Basil

TURMERIC
Curcuma longa, Curcuma domestica, Curcuma aromatica Herbal remedy.

Indications: Orally – for amenorrhoea, premenstrual syndrome, pruritus, indigestion, abdominal pain, diarrhoea, flatulence, abdominal bloating, loss of appetite, oedema, cystitis, stress. Also for arthritis, inflammatory gastrointestinal disorders, *Helicobacter pylori* infection, hepatobiliary conditions, bronchitis, postoperative pain, depression, joint pain. Topically – for pain relief, sprains, bruising, eye infections, inflammatory skin conditions, psoriasis, periodontitis, gingivitis.

Safety in pregnancy: Appears safe in amounts commonly used in foods and in small amounts topically. AVOID THERAPEUTIC ORAL DOSES IN PREGNANCY – may cause uterine contractions, leading to miscarriage, preterm labour, hypertonic uterine action. Appears safe orally and topically when breastfeeding.

Contraindications and precautions: Iron deficiency anaemia, gall bladder disease, gallstones, haemorrhagic and coagulation disorders, diabetes mellitus, oesophageal reflux disease, hormone-sensitive conditions, infertility.

Adverse effects: Orally – constipation, indigestion, diarrhoea, distension, gastroesophageal reflux, nausea, vomiting, pruritus, pitting oedema. Topically – allergic contact dermatitis, urticaria, pruritus.

Interactions: Therapeutic oral doses, prolonged, excessive or inappropriate use may interact with anticoagulants and antiplatelet drugs: heparin, warfarin, aspirin, diclofenac, ibuprofen, enoxaparin. Also antidiabetic medication, theophylline, pentazocine, propranolol, fentanyl, lignocaine, oestrogens, cimetidine, ranitidine, antifungal agents, erythromycin. Herbs: angelica, clove, devil's claw, fenugreek, feverfew, garlic, ginger, ginkgo, meadowsweet, Panax ginseng, psyllium, red clover, Siberian ginseng, turmeric, willow.

UMCHAMO WEMFENE *see* Baboon urine

UMCKALOABO
Pelargonium sidoides Herbal remedy, also known as African geranium.

Indications: Orally – for bronchitis, sinusitis, pharyngitis, tonsillitis, common cold; herpes, tuberculosis, gonorrhoea, dysentery, diarrhoea.

Safety in pregnancy: No evidence of safety in pregnancy and breastfeeding; contains anticoagulant coumarins – advise caution.

Contraindications and precautions: Avoid with threatened miscarriage, antepartum haemorrhage, low-lying placenta or placenta praevia; advise caution with heavy lochia, particularly if retained products of conception. Avoid with autoimmune diseases – may be immunostimulant. Avoid with haemorrhagic disorders.

Adverse effects: Diarrhoea, allergic skin reactions; pyrexia, tachycardia, bruising, bleeding.

Interactions: Therapeutic oral doses, prolonged, excessive or inappropriate use may interact with anticoagulants and antiplatelet drugs: heparin, warfarin, aspirin, diclofenac, ibuprofen, enoxaparin. Also antihypertensives, immunosuppressants. Anticoagulant herbs: angelica, clove, fenugreek, feverfew, garlic, ginger, ginkgo, meadowsweet, Panax ginseng, red clover, turmeric, willow bark.

UVA URSI
Arctostaphylos uva-ursi, Arbutus uva-ursi Herbal remedy, also known as Bearberry.

Indications: Orally – for cystitis, urinary tract infections, as a diuretic, dysuria, pyelonephritis, benign prostatic hyperplasia, constipation, bronchitis.

Safety in pregnancy: AVOID THERAPEUTIC ORAL DOSES IN PREGNANCY – may have oxytocic effects, causing miscarriage, preterm labour;

may be mutagenic, carcinogenic. Advise caution: insufficient information on safety when breastfeeding.

Contraindications and precautions: Avoid with renal and hepatic disease, hypertension, Crohn's disease, other inflammatory bowel conditions, conditions causing thinning of retina.

Adverse effects: Orally – long-term use can cause nausea, vomiting, tinnitus, insomnia, irritability, dyspnoea, cyanosis, convulsions, death. May cause greenish-brown discolouration of urine.

Interactions: Therapeutic oral doses, prolonged, excessive or inappropriate use may interact with progesterone, diazepam, potassium phosphate, iron therapy, non-steroidal anti-inflammatory drugs, corticosteroids. Herbs: none identified.

VALERIAN
Valeriana officinalis Herbal remedy.

Indications: Orally – for insomnia, dysmenorrhoea, premenstrual syndrome, menopausal symptoms. Also for depression, anxiety, stress, chronic fatigue syndrome; muscle and joint pain, infantile convulsions, attention deficit-hyperactivity disorder. Topically – for sleep disorders.

Safety in pregnancy: Little information available, but conflicting opinions on safety in pregnancy – advise caution. Animal research suggests may cause reduced zinc levels in fetal brain.

Contraindications and precautions: Avoid prior to surgery to reduce risk of central nervous system depression.

Adverse effects: Headache, insomnia, vivid dreams, dry mouth, gastrointestinal disturbance, excitability, cardiac issues. Prolonged use may cause withdrawal symptoms on discontinuation.

Interactions: Therapeutic oral doses, prolonged, excessive or inappropriate use may interact with oestrogens, oral contraceptives, alcohol, benzodiazepines, central nervous system depressants, anaesthetics. Sedative herbs: California poppy, catnip, hops, Jamaican dogwood, kava, St John's wort, skullcap.

VERBENA
Verbena officinalis Herbal remedy, also known as Blue vervain.

Indications: Orally – for menopausal complaints, irregular menstruation, increasing lactation, pain relief. Also for sore throat, asthma, whooping cough, depression, hysteria, exhaustion, diseases of liver, gall bladder, renal and gastrointestinal tracts, gout, anaemia, oedema. Topically – for wound healing, abscesses, burns, arthritis, rheumatism, bruising, itching, minor burns.

Safety in pregnancy: Caution: insufficient information on safety in pregnancy.

Contraindications and precautions: Any compromised pregnancy, labour, postnatal physiology; iron deficiency anaemia. Do not confuse with lemon verbena (*Aloysia citrodora*).

Adverse effects: Contact dermatitis and hypersensitivity.

Interactions: Therapeutic oral doses, prolonged, excessive or inappropriate use may interact with barbiturates, iron therapy. Herbs: none identified.

VITEX AGNUS CASTUS

Vitex agnus castus Herbal remedy, also known as Chaste berry, Chaste tree.

Indications: Orally – for dysmenorrhoea, secondary amenorrhoea, metrorrhagia, oligomenorrhea, menopausal symptoms, premenstrual syndrome, female infertility, progesterone insufficiency, postpartum vaginal bleeding; bleeding associated with intrauterine contraceptive device, for retained placenta, to stimulate lactation. Also to promote micturition, to reduce excessive libido, for acne, anxiety, common cold, headache, insomnia, fracture, oedema. Topically – for insect bites, stings.

Safety in pregnancy: AVOID ORAL USE IN PRECONCEPTION PERIOD, PREGNANCY AND BREASTFEEDING – hormonal effects may compromise implantation, pregnancy, lactation. Topical use appears safe.

Contraindications and precautions: Avoid with hormone-sensitive conditions, for example endometriosis, uterine fibroids, ovarian and breast cancer. Advise women about to undergo ovarian stimulation therapy for infertility to inform doctor, avoid concomitant use with bromocriptine and other drugs to stimulate ovulation; discontinue use before ovarian stimulation – risk of ovarian hyperstimulation syndrome, possibly fatal. Avoid with schizophrenia.

Adverse effects: Skin itching, stomach cramps, diarrhoea, nausea, vomiting, headache, fatigue, insomnia, irregular menstruation.

Interactions: Therapeutic oral doses, prolonged, excessive or inappropriate use may interact with hormone replacement therapy, contraceptive Pill, bromocriptine, metoclopramide, chlorpromazine, prochlorperazine, levodopa. Oestrogenic herbs: black cohosh, blue cohosh, dong quai, evening primrose, fennel, fenugreek, ginkgo, ginseng, liquorice, raspberry leaf, red clover.

WHEATGRASS

Triticum aestivum Herbal remedy.

Indications: Orally – for iron deficiency anaemia, wound healing, urinary tract infections, hypertension, hypercholesterolaemia, diabetes mellitus, renal calculi; to aid metabolism of drugs, liver and circulatory detoxification. Topically – for chronic skin conditions, rheumatic pain.

Safety in pregnancy: Appears safe in amounts commonly used in foods. Caution: insufficient evidence available to confirm safety of therapeutic doses in pregnancy.

Contraindications and precautions: May lower blood glucose, caution in diabetes mellitus.

Adverse effects: Nausea, anorexia, constipation.

Interactions: Therapeutic oral doses, prolonged, excessive or inappropriate use may interact with antidiabetic drugs. Hypoglycaemic herbs: bitter melon, devil's claw, fenugreek, garlic, horse chestnut, Panax ginseng, psyllium, Siberian ginseng.

WILD DAGGA *see* Motherwort

WILD DAISY
Bellis perennis Herbal remedy.

Indications: Orally – for coughs, bronchitis, hepatic and renal disorders, inflammation, as an expectorant, astringent. Topically – for wounds, skin diseases, to slow bleeding.

Safety in pregnancy: Advise caution: insufficient information on safety in pregnancy. In view of purported effect in slowing bleeding, caution advised at term when clotting factors increase.

Contraindications and precautions: Do not confuse with homeopathic *Bellis perennis*. Keep fresh flowers, medicinal products away from cats – toxic.

Adverse effects: Allergic reactions especially if sensitive to the Asteraceae/Compositae plant family – ragweed, chrysanthemums, marigolds, daisies.

Interactions: None documented.

WILD MARJORAM *see* Oregano

WILD YAM
Dioscorea alata Herbal remedy.

Indications: Orally – for menopausal vaginal dryness, premenstrual syndrome, menstrual disorders, infertility, contraception, to increase libido. Topically – for menopausal hot flushes, menstrual disorders, infertility.

Safety in pregnancy: AVOID THERAPEUTIC ORAL AND TOPICAL USE IN PREGNANCY – phytoestrogens may cause miscarriage, preterm labour.

Contraindications and precautions: Avoid with oestrogens, progesterone, hormone replacement therapy. Avoid with hormone-sensitive conditions – breast, uterine and ovarian cancer, endometriosis, fibroids. Avoid with conditions that increase risk of thrombosis.

Adverse effects: Nausea, vomiting, headache.

Interactions: Therapeutic oral doses, prolonged, excessive or inappropriate use may interact with oestrogens, contraceptive Pill, hormone replacement therapy. Oestrogenic herbs: black cohosh, blue cohosh, dong quai, evening primrose, fennel, fenugreek, ginkgo, ginseng, liquorice, raspberry leaf, red clover, vitex agnus castus.

WILLOW BARK
Salix alba Herbal remedy.

Indications: Orally – for dysmenorrhoea, headache, pain, as an anti-inflammatory, for arthritis, gout, common cold, influenza. Willow also available as liquid Bach Flower Rescue Remedy taken orally, diluted in spring water, for doubt and negative outlook.

Safety in pregnancy: AVOID THERAPEUTIC ORAL USE IN PREGNANCY unless under the supervision of a qualified medical herbalist – salicylates may cause bleeding, miscarriage. AVOID ORAL USE DURING BREAST FEEDING – salicylates excreted in breast milk, increase risk of bleeding. Bach Flower Rescue Remedy appears safe.

Contraindications and precautions: Avoid with prophylactic aspirin, enoxaparin or other prophylactic drugs in pregnancy. Avoid with pre-existing sensitivity to aspirin. Avoid with haemorrhagic disorders; threatened miscarriage, antepartum, postpartum haemorrhage; renal conditions. Discontinue at least two weeks prior to elective surgery. Avoid Bach Flower Rescue Remedy with liver disease, alcohol dependency, severe mental health issues.

Adverse effects: Gastric irritation, colitis; itching, allergic reactions. Unstable blood pressure; reduction in renal perfusion. Risk of anaphylaxis, especially if allergic to aspirin.

Interactions: Therapeutic oral doses, prolonged, excessive or inappropriate use may interact with anticoagulants and antiplatelet drugs: heparin, warfarin, aspirin, diclofenac, ibuprofen, enoxaparin. Anticoagulant herbs: angelica, clove, fenugreek, feverfew, garlic, ginger, ginkgo, meadowsweet, Panax ginseng, poplar, red clover, turmeric, willow.

WIND FLOWER *see* Pulsatilla

WINTERGREEN
Gaultheria procumbens Herbal remedy, also known as Deerberry.

Indications: Orally – for dysmenorrhoea, headache, abdominal pain, flatulence, fever, kidney stones, asthma, sciatica and backache, rheumatoid arthritis. Topically – for muscle soreness, back pain, as an antiseptic.

Safety in pregnancy: AVOID ORAL AND TOPICAL USE IN PREGNANCY, LABOUR, BREASTFEEDING – contains toxic methyl salicylate.

Contraindications and precautions: Salicylate allergy, gastric ulcers and inflammation.

Adverse effects: Orally – salicylate poisoning – tinnitus, nausea, vomiting, diarrhoea, headache, stomach pain, confusion. Topically – skin irritation.

Interactions: Therapeutic oral doses, prolonged, excessive or inappropriate use may interact with aspirin, warfarin and anticoagulant herbs: angelica, fenugreek, feverfew, garlic, ginger, ginkgo, meadowsweet, Panax ginseng, red clover, turmeric, willow bark.

WITCH HAZEL

Hamamelis virginiana Herbal remedy.

Indications: Orally – for diarrhoea, colitis, haematemesis, common cold. Topically – for acne, itching, skin inflammation or injury, mucous membrane inflammation, varicose veins, haemorrhoids, bruises, insect bites, minor burns, as an astringent and haemostatic for wounds, itching, haemorrhoids, teething, insect bites. Tannin content thought to reduce wound irritation and inflammation, bleeding and to draw wound edges together. Popular treatment for perineal healing post-delivery.

Safety in pregnancy: Appears safe to use topically, well diluted, in pregnancy and postnatal period. AVOID THERAPEUTIC ORAL USE IN PREGNANCY AND BREASTFEEDING – contains very small amounts of carcinogenic safrole, as well as tannins which, in large doses, can be hepatotoxic.

Contraindications and precautions: Avoid topical use on perineum if wound becomes inflamed, infected.

Adverse effects: Orally – gastrointestinal disturbance, renal and hepatic damage; topically – contact dermatitis, redness, burning.

Interactions: None documented.

WOLF'S CLAW *see* Club moss

YAM *see* Wild yam

YARROW

Achillea millefolium, Achillea borealis Herbal remedy, also known as Bloodwort.

Indications: Orally – for amenorrhoea, colds, allergic rhinitis, toothache; diarrhoea, irritable bowel syndrome; to induce sweating. Topically – for gingivitis, bleeding haemorrhoids, wound healing.

Safety in pregnancy: AVOID ORAL AND TOPICAL USE IN PREGNANCY – contains thujone, abortifacient. Caution: insufficient safety evidence on breastfeeding.

Contraindications and precautions: Avoid with excessive lochial bleeding, retained products of conception, haemorrhagic or coagulation disorders. Avoid with allergy to plants in the Asteraceae/Compositae family including ragweed, chrysanthemums, marigolds, daisies. Do not confuse with Bloodroot.

Adverse effects: Orally in large amounts – sedative and diuretic effects. Topically – allergic dermatitis. Orally, large amounts of yarrow might cause sedative effects.

Interactions: Therapeutic oral doses, prolonged, excessive or inappropriate use may interact with anticoagulants and antiplatelet drugs: heparin, warfarin, aspirin, diclofenac, ibuprofen, enoxaparin. Also antacids, cimetidine, ranitidine, lithium. Anticoagulant herbs: angelica, fenugreek, feverfew, garlic, ginger, ginkgo, meadowsweet, Panax ginseng, turmeric, willow bark.

YELLOW HORSE *see* Ma huang

YELLOW JASMINE *see* Gelsemium, herbal remedy, homeopathic remedy

YERBA MATE

Ilex paraguariensis Herbal remedy, also known as Chimarrao.

Indications: Orally – for chronic fatigue, depression, headache; joint pain, osteoporosis; diabetes and pre-diabetes; hypotension, renal calculi, urinary tract infection, as a laxative. Popular beverage in Latin and South America.

Safety in pregnancy: AVOID ORAL CONSUMPTION, INCLUDING TEA, IN PREGNANCY – high caffeine content may cause miscarriage, preterm labour, low birth weight. AVOID DURING BREASTFEEDING – caffeine content may cause neonatal irritability, diarrhoea.

Contraindications and precautions: Avoid excessive or prolonged ingestion – caffeine content may have carcinogenic effect. Do not confuse with yerba mansa (*Anemia californica*).

Adverse effects: Significant evidence of carcinogenicity; insomnia, headache, tachycardia, hyperventilation, cardiac arrhythmias, increased diuresis, nausea, vomiting. Abrupt withdrawal after prolonged consumption may cause irritation, dizziness, anxiety.

Interactions: Therapeutic oral doses, prolonged, excessive or inappropriate use may interact with anticoagulants and antiplatelet drugs: heparin, warfarin, aspirin, diclofenac, ibuprofen, enoxaparin. Also antidiabetic medication, certain antibiotics, amphetamines, alcohol, benzodiazepines, carbamazepine, cimetidine, cocaine, calcium supplements, magnesium, contraceptive Pill, oestrogens, hormone replacement therapy, fluconazole, lithium, monoamine oxidase inhibitors, nicotine, phenobarbitone, phenytoin, verapamil. Anticoagulant herbs: angelica, clove, fenugreek, feverfew, garlic, ginger, ginkgo, meadowsweet, Panax ginseng, poplar, red clover, turmeric, willow. Hypoglycaemic herbs: bitter melon, cinnamon, ginger, ginseng, milk thistle. Oestrogenic herbs: black cohosh, blue cohosh, dong quai, evening primrose, fennel, fenugreek, ginkgo, ginseng, liquorice, raspberry leaf, red clover, vitex agnus castus.

YLANG YLANG

Cananga odorata Herbal remedy.

Indications: Topically, essential oil in aromatherapy – as a relaxant, sedative, hypotensive, aphrodisiac, indirect analgesic; for stress, fear, anxiety; insomnia, fatigue, to reduce blood pressure, ease muscular pain, to aid recovery from birth. Also antiseptic, antibacterial, antifungal.

Safety in pregnancy: Essential oil appears safe topically and by inhalation in doses up to 1.5% in pregnancy, 2% in labour and postnatal period.

Contraindications and precautions: Avoid in individuals with moderate to severe clinical depression, especially if on antidepressant medication: anecdotal evidence suggests its deep sedative effects may exacerbate introspective tendencies. Caution with postural/supine hypotension, epidural anaesthesia due to significant hypotensive effect. Beware effect on women prone to hay fever and asthma triggered by flower pollen – possible psychosomatic effect. Do not confuse with cananga oil. Do not ingest. Do not use neat on skin or directly in a birthing pool. Use a diffuser for a maximum of 15–20 minutes in any hour; do not vaporize in the second stage of labour to avoid neonatal exposure; do not diffuse near neonates, elderly or ill people. Do not diffuse near animals – toxic to cats and dogs. Do not diffuse in public areas or use excessive amounts which spread to public areas of maternity unit, to avoid excessive exposure of the woman, baby, visitors and staff to potential adverse effects. Discontinue use if any allergic reactions occur to avoid accumulative reaction to specific chemicals – may lead to anaphylactic shock in severe cases. May be adulterated with cheaper oils – adulterated oil becomes cloudy. Store in a refrigerator; do not use with or store near homeopathic remedies.

Adverse effects: Topically – contact dermatitis. By inhalation – can have sedative effect or cause loss of concentration in staff. Overpowering aroma may cause nausea, headache.

Interactions: Therapeutic oral doses may interact with antihypotensive drugs and herbs: flaxseed, garlic, ginger, hawthorn, lavender.

YOHIMBE

Pausinystalia yohimbe Herbal remedy.

Indications: Orally – as an aphrodisiac, hallucinogen; for erectile dysfunction, sexual dysfunction in men and women, to aid athletic performance, for weight loss, exhaustion, hypertension, diabetic neuropathy. Commonly used in African medicine.

Safety in pregnancy: AVOID THERAPEUTIC ORAL USE IN PREGNANCY OR BREASTFEEDING – possible fetal toxicity and uterine hypotonia.

Contraindications and precautions: Advise caution unless under the supervision of an appropriately qualified medical practitioner. Do not use for children.

Adverse effects: Nausea, vomiting, diarrhoea; decreased libido, muscle aches; dizziness, headache, vertigo; hypotension, tachycardia, oedema, cardiac arrhythmia, myocardial infarction due to yohimbine content; insomnia, anxiety, agitation, exacerbation of pre-existing mental ill health.

Interactions: Therapeutic oral doses, prolonged, excessive or inappropriate use may interact with anticoagulants and antiplatelet drugs: heparin, warfarin, aspirin, diclofenac, ibuprofen, enoxaparin. Also amitriptyline, clozapine, codeine, fentanyl, fluoxetine, methadone; monoamine oxidase inhibitors, naloxone, phenothiazines, stimulants, tricyclic antidepressants. Herbs: berberine and caffeine-containing products and herbs; ma huang. Also anticoagulant herbs: angelica, fenugreek, feverfew, garlic, ginger, ginkgo, meadowsweet, Panax ginseng, turmeric, willow. Tyramine-containing foods such as cheese; also fava beans, cola, chocolate.

YUCCA

Yucca aloifolia, *Yucca brevifolia* Herbal remedy, also known as Aloe yucca, Dagger plant.

Indications: Orally – for hypertension, migraines, poor circulation; colitis, other gastric conditions; diabetes, osteoarthritis, hepatic and gall bladder disorders. Root cooked and eaten in certain cultures to cleanse blood. Topically – for sore, inflamed skin, bleeding, sprains, broken limbs, joint pain, baldness, dandruff.

Safety in pregnancy: Appears safe in amounts commonly used in foods. Advise caution: insufficient information on safety of therapeutic oral use in pregnancy.

Contraindications and precautions: Avoid with any medical or obstetric conditions; avoid with skin conditions, hay fever. Plant toxic to dogs. Do not confuse with Aloe vera. Do not confuse with cassava (*Manihot esculenta*, also known as yuca) – sometimes used to induce labour, but contains toxic, teratogenic cyanic glycosides when unprocessed.

Adverse effects: Contact dermatitis, itching; allergic rhinitis, hay fever.

Interactions: None documented.

Glossary of Terms

Abortifacient	Capable of causing miscarriage
Acidosis	Increased acid in the blood
Alopecia	Hair loss
Amenorrhoea	Absence of menstruation, as with pregnancy
Amitriptyline	Antidepressant drug
Amoxycillin	Antibiotic drug, part of penicillin group
Anticholinergics	Drugs that block action of acetylcholine
Antihypertensives	Drugs that reduce blood pressure
Antiplatelets	Drugs that inhibit thrombus formation
Aromatase inhibitors	Drugs used for breast cancer in postmenopausal women
Benzodiazepines	Sedative drugs, not commonly used in pregnancy
Bradycardia	A slow heart rate
Bupivacaine	Pain-relieving drug used in epidural anaesthesia
Calcium channel blockers	Drugs to reduce blood pressure, irregular heart rhythm
Calculi	Stones, as in kidney or gallstones
Caput succedaneum	Oedema (swelling) seen on baby's head at birth, usually resulting from difficult birth
Carbamazepine	Anticonvulsant and analgesic drug
Carcinogenic	Causes cancer

Central nervous system depressants	Sedative, tranquillizing, hypnotic drugs
Cimetidine	Drug for heartburn and gastrointestinal ulcers
Clozapine	Antipsychotic drug
Colitis	Inflammation of colon in digestive tract
Cyanogenic glycosides	Naturally occurring plant toxins
Cyclosporine	Immunosuppressive drug to prevent transplant rejection
Diazepam	Calming drug, part of benzodiazepine family
Diclofenac	Non-steroidal anti-inflammatory drug to treat pain, inflammation
Digoxin	Drug to regulate heart rate and rhythm, not commonly used in pregnancy
Dinoprostone	Prostaglandin E2 used for labour induction and postpartum haemorrhage
Diuretic	Drug that increases urination
Dysmenorrhoea	Painful menstrual periods
Dyspnoea	Difficulty breathing
Dysuria	Difficulty in passing urine
Emmenagoguic	Capable of causing menstruation-like vaginal bleeding
Enoxaparin	Anticoagulant drug
Enuresis	Bedwetting
Epistaxis	Nosebleed
Estragole	Essential oil chemical with aniseed-like aroma, may be carcinogenic, toxic
Excoriation	Scraped skin
Expectorant	Promotes secretion of sputum
Fentanyl	Opioid analgesic
Flavonoids	Antioxidant plant pigments
Fluconazole	Antifungal drug
Fluoxetine	Antidepressant, also known as Prozac™
Fluvastatin	Statin drug to reduce high cholesterol
Furanocoumarins	Potentially toxic chemical compounds found in some plants
Galactorrhoea	Excessive milk production

Gingivitis	Inflammation of gums
Glucocorticoids	Anti-inflammatory corticosteroids
Glucose 6 phosphate dehydrogenase (G6PD) deficiency	Hereditary haemolytic condition, lack of G6PD enzyme
Gynaecomastia	Enlargement of male breasts, usually hormonal imbalance
Haematuria	Blood in urine
Heparin	Anticoagulant drug
Hepatobiliary	Pertaining to liver and gall bladder
Hepatotoxic	Toxic to liver
Hypercholesterolaemia	Excessive cholesterol in blood
Hyperemesis gravidarum	Excessive vomiting in pregnancy, with weight loss and dehydration
Hyperlipidaemia	Excessive fats in blood
Hyperpyrexia	Excessive body temperature
Hypertension	High blood pressure
Hypertonic	Excessive action as in uterine contractions
Hypoglycaemia	Low blood glucose
Hypokalaemia	Low potassium in blood
Hyponatraemia	Excessively low salt levels in the blood
Hypotension	Low blood pressure
Imipramine	Antidepressant drug
Involution	Shrinking of organ, as in uterus after childbirth
Isoniazid	Bacteriostatic drug, primarily used for tuberculosis
Kernicterus	Brain damage due to excessive jaundice in newborn
Lithium	Drug for bipolar disorder
Lochia	Blood loss after labour
Loperamide	Drug to reduce intestinal movement
Maple syrup urine disease	Inherited metabolic disorder, infant's urine has odour of maple syrup
Mastalgia	Breast pain
Menorrhagia	Excessive menstrual bleeding
Methyldopa	Antihypertensive drug

Monoamine oxidase inhibitors	Antidepressant drugs
Mutagenic	Liable to cause genetic mutations
Neonate	Newborn baby up to the age of four weeks
Niacin	Nicotinic acid, part of vitamin B complex
Obstetric cholestasis	Liver condition in pregnancy, causes skin itching
Ondansetron	Drug for nausea and vomiting
Oestradiol	Oestrogen-type steroid hormone, female sex hormone
Oxidation/oxidization	In essential oil, deterioration caused by exposure to oxygen
Oxytocic	Drug used to expedite labour
Pentazocine	Analgesic used in labour
Phaechromocytoma	Rare adrenal gland tumour
Phenobarbital	Narcotic, sedative drug, used in epilepsy
Phenothiazines	Tranquillizing drugs used for some mental health issues
Phenytoin	Anticonvulsant drug used in epilepsy
Photosensitivity	Sensitivity to sunlight
Phytoestrogens	Plant substances with hormonal action
Placental abruption	Separation of placenta in pregnancy
Pneumonitis	Inflammation of lungs
Precipitate labour	Rapid labour, usually less than three hours' duration
Prophylactic	Preventative
Propranolol	Beta blocker, used for cardiac arrythmia
Proteinuria	Protein in the urine, a sign of pre-eclampsia in pregnancy
Raynaud's syndrome	Circulatory disorder characterized by cold extremities
Selective serotonin reuptake inhibitors (SSRIs)	Antidepressants used for major depression, anxiety
Systemic lupus erythematosus	Autoimmune condition affecting joints, skin, kidneys, other organs
Tachycardia	Excessive heart rate/pulse

Tamoxifen	Breast cancer drug
Tannins	Plant chemicals with unpleasant taste, to deter animals eating unripe fruit or seeds
Teratogenic	Relating to, or causing, embryonic malformations
Theophylline	Drug used for asthma
Tramadol	Opioid analgesic for moderate to severe pain
Urticaria	Skin redness, inflammation, swelling, usually due to allergic reaction
Uterine polarity	Physiological balance between upper and lower segments of uterus
Uterotonic	Substance that stimulates uterine contractions
Venepuncture	Insertion of needle into a vein to draw blood
Verapamil	Drug for cardiac arrythmias and kidney conditions
Warfarin	Anticoagulant drug
Wernicke's encephalopathy	Life-threatening vitamin B1 deficiency

References

Abbassi, J. (2017) 'Amid reports of infant deaths, FTC cracks down on homeopathy while FDA investigates.' *JAMA Network* 28 February. Available at http://jamanetwork.com/journals/jama/article-abstract/2602995

Abebe, W. (2019) 'Review of herbal medications with the potential to cause bleeding: Dental implications, and risk prediction and prevention avenues.' *EPMA Journal* 10(1), 51–64.

Abedzadeh-Kalahroudi, M. (2014) 'Complementary and alternative medicine in midwifery.' *Nursing and Midwifery Studies 3*(2), e19449.

Abinavhavi, T.M. (2014) 'Homeopathy – India's traditional system of medicine.' *Nikkei Asian Review* 6 March. Available at https://asia.nikkei.com/Business/Technology/Homeopathy-India-s-traditional-system-of-medicine

Adane, F., Seyoum, G., Alamneh, Y.M., Abie, W., Desta, M. and Sisay, B. (2020) 'Herbal medicine use and predictors among pregnant women attending antenatal care in Ethiopia: A systematic review and meta-analysis.' *BMC Pregnancy Childbirth 20*, 157.

Adib-Hajbaghery, M. and Hoseinian, M. (2014) 'Knowledge, attitude and practice toward complementary and traditional medicine among Kashan health care staff.' *Complementary Therapies in Medicine 22*(1), 126–132.

Ahmed, M., Hwang, J.H., Choi, S. and Han, D. (2017) 'Safety classification of herbal medicines used among pregnant women in Asian countries: A systematic review.' *BMC Complementary and Alternative Medicine 17*, 489.

Ahmed, M., Hwang, J.H., Hasan, M.A. and Han, D. (2018) 'Herbal medicine use by pregnant women in Bangladesh: A cross-sectional study.' *BMC Complementary and Alternative Medicine 18*(1), 333.

Ahmed, S.M., Nordeng, H., Sundby, J., Aragaw, Y.A. and de Boer, H.J. (2018) 'The use of medicinal plants by pregnant women in Africa: A systematic review.' *Journal of Ethnopharmacology 224*, 297–313.

Akour, A., Kasabri, V., Afifi, F.U. and Bulatova, N. (2016) 'The use of medicinal herbs in gynecological and pregnancy-related disorders by Jordanian women: A review of folkloric practice vs. evidence-based pharmacology.' *Pharmaceutical Biology 54*(9), 1901–1918.

Al Essa, M., Alissa, A., Alanizi, A., Bustami, R., *et al.* (2019) 'Pregnant women's use and attitude toward herbal, vitamin, and mineral supplements in an academic tertiary care center, Riyadh, Saudi Arabia.' *Saudi Pharmaceutical Journal 27*(1), 138–144.

Ali-Shtayeh, M.S., Jamous, R.M. and Jamous, R.M. (2015) 'Plants used during pregnancy, childbirth, postpartum and infant healthcare in Palestine.' *Complementary Therapies in Clinical Practice 21*(2), 84–93.

Allen, E.N., Gomes, M., Yevoo, L., Egesah, O., *et al.* (2014) 'Influences on participant reporting in the World Health Organisation drugs exposure pregnancy registry: A qualitative study.' *BMC Health Services Research 14*, 525.

Alonso-Castro, A.J. (2014) 'Use of medicinal fauna in Mexican traditional medicine.' *Journal of Ethnopharmacology 152*(1), 53–70.

Andrade, R.J., Medina-Caliz, I., Gonzalez-Jimenez, A., Garcia-Cortes, M. and Lucena, M.I. (2018) 'Hepatic damage by natural remedies.' *Seminars in Liver Disease 38*(1), 21–40.

Angelon-Gaetz, K.A., Klaus, C., Chaudhry, E.A. and Bean, D.K. (2018) 'Lead in spices, herbal remedies, and ceremonial powders sampled from home investigations for children with elevated blood lead levels – North Carolina, 2011–2018.' US Department of Health and Human Services/Centers for Disease Control and Prevention. *Morbidity and Mortality Weekly Report (MMWR) 67*(46).

Apaydin, E.A., Maher, A.R., Shanman, R., Booth, M.S., *et al.* (2016) 'A systematic review of St John's wort for major depressive disorder.' *Systematic Reviews 5*, 148. Available at https://systematicreviewsjournal.biomedcentral.com/articles/10.1186/s13643-016-0325-2#citeas

Arabiat, D.H., Whitehead, L., Al Jabery, M., Towell-Barnard, A., Shields, L. and Abu Sabah, E. (2019) 'Traditional methods for managing illness in newborns and infants in an Arab society.' *International Nursing Review 66*(3), 329–337.

Asif, M. (2012) 'A brief study of toxic effects of some medicinal herbs on kidney.' *Advanced Biomedical Research 1*, 44.

Assmann, C.E., Cadoná, F.C., Bonadiman, B.D.S.R., Dornelles, E.B., Trevisan, G. and Cruz, I.B.M.D. (2018) 'Tea tree oil presents in vitro antitumor activity on breast cancer cells without cytotoxic effects on fibroblasts and on peripheral blood mononuclear cells.' *Biomedicine & Pharmacotherapy 103*, 1253–1261.

ATMS (Australian Traditional Medicines Society) (2018) 'Australians turn to natural therapies in the millions.' Media release 17 May. Available at www.atms.com.au/wp-content/uploads/2018/10/Australians-turn-to-natural-therapies-in-the-millions-FINAL.pdf?x85875

Awad, A. and Al-Shaye, D. (2014) 'Public awareness, patterns of use and attitudes toward natural health products in Kuwait: A cross-sectional survey.' *BMC Complementary and Alternative Medicine 14*, 105.

Awortwe, C., Makiwane, M., Reuter, H., Muller, C., Louw, J. and Rosenkranz, B. (2018) 'Critical evaluation of causality assessment of herb–drug interactions in patients.' *British Journal of Clinical Pharmacology 84*, 679–693.

Aziato, L. and Omenyo, C.N. (2018) 'Initiation of traditional birth attendants and their traditional and spiritual practices during pregnancy and childbirth in Ghana.' *BMC Pregnancy and Childbirth 18*(64). Available at www.ncbi.nlm.nih.gov/pmc/articles/PMC5842514

Bahall, M. (2017) 'Use of complementary and alternative medicine by patients with end-stage renal disease on haemodialysis in Trinidad: A descriptive study.' *BMC Complementary and Alternative Medicine 17*(1), 250.

Ball, P. (2004) 'The memory of water.' *Nature.* Available at www.nature.com/news/2004/041004/full/news041004-19.html

Barišić, T., Pecirep, A., Milićević, R., Vasilj, A. and Tirić, D. (2017) 'What do pregnant women know about harmful effects of medication and herbal remedies use during pregnancy?' *Psychiatria Danubina 29*(Suppl. 4), 804–811.

Barnes, L.A.J., Barclay, L., McCaffery, K. and Aslani, P. (2018) 'Complementary medicine products used in pregnancy and lactation and an examination of the information sources accessed pertaining to maternal health literacy: A systematic review of qualitative studies.' *BMC Complementary and Alternative Medicine 18*(1), 229.

Benjamins, L.J., Gourishankar, A., Yataco-Marquez, V., Cardona, E.H. and de Ybarrondo, L. (2013) 'Honey pacifier use among an indigent pediatric population.' *Pediatrics 131*(6), e1838–e1841.

Bettiol, A., Lombardi, N., Marconi, E., Crescioli, G., *et al.* (2018) 'The use of complementary and alternative medicines during breastfeeding: Results from the Herbal supplements in Breastfeeding InvesTigation (HaBIT) study.' *British Journal of Clinical Pharmacology 84*(9), 2040–2047.

Birdee, G.S., Kemper, K.J., Rothman, R. and Gardiner, P. (2014) 'Use of complementary and alternative medicine during pregnancy and the postpartum period: An analysis of the National Health Interview Survey.' *Journal of Women's Health (Larchmt) 23*(10), 824–829.

Bolhuis, K., Kushner, S.A., Yalniz, S., Hillegers, M.H.J., *et al.* (2018) 'Maternal and paternal cannabis use during pregnancy and the risk of psychotic-like experiences in the offspring.' *Schizophrenia Research 202*, 322–327.

Boltman-Binkowski, H. (2016) 'A systematic review: Are herbal and homeopathic remedies used during pregnancy safe?' *Curationis 39*(1), 1514.

Bone, K. (2012) 'Are auto-immune herbs safe during auto-immune disease?' *Dynamic Chiropractic 30*, 17. Available at www.dynamicchiropractic.com/mpacms/dc/article.php?id=56063

Brantley, S.J., Argikar, A.A., Lin, Y.S., Nagar, S. and Paine, M.F. (2014) 'Herb–drug interactions: Challenges and opportunities for improved predictions.' *Drug Metabolism & Disposition 42*(3), 301–317.

Bruno, L.O., Simoes, R.S., de Jesus Simoes, M., Girão, M.J.B.C. and Grundmann, O. (2018) 'Pregnancy and herbal medicines: An unnecessary risk for women's health – A narrative review.' *Phytotherapy Research 32*(5), 796–810.

Cardoso, B.S. and Amaral, V.C.S. (2019) 'The use of phytotherapy during pregnancy: A global overview.' *Cien Saude Colet 24*(4), 1439–1450.

Carvalho, A.C., Ramalho, L.S., Marques, R.F. and Perfeito, J.P. (2014) 'Regulation of herbal medicines in Brazil.' *Journal of Ethnopharmacology 158*, Pt B, 503–506.

Chakravorty, J., Meyer-Rochow, V.B. and Ghosh, S. (2011) 'Vertebrates used for medicinal purposes by members of the Nyishi and Galo tribes in Arunachal Pradesh (North-East India).' *Journal of Ethnobiology and Ethnomedicine 7*, 13. Available at www.ncbi.nlm.nih.gov/pmc/articles/PMC3079603

Cho, Y.M., Kwon, J.E., Lee, M., Lea, Y., *et al.* (2018) '*Agrimonia eupatoria L.* (Agrimony) extract alters liver health in subjects with elevated alanine transaminase levels: A controlled, randomized, and double-blind trial.' *Journal of Medicinal Food 21*(3), 282–288.

Choi, S., Oh, D.-S. and Jerng, U.M. (2017) 'A systematic review of the pharmacokinetic and pharmacodynamic interactions of herbal medicine with warfarin.' *PLoS One 12*(8), e0182794. Available at www.ncbi.nlm.nih.gov/pmc/articles/PMC5552262

Clarke, T.C., Black, L.I., Stussman, B.J., Barnes, P.M. and Nahin, R.L. (2015) 'Trends in the use of complementary health approaches among adults: United States, 2002–2012.' *National Health Statistics Reports 10*(79), 1–16.

Close, C., Sinclair, M., McCullough, J.E., Liddle, S.D. and Hughes, C.M. (2016) 'Factors affecting recruitment and attrition in randomised controlled trials of complementary and alternative medicine for pregnancy-related issues.' *Evidence-Based Complementary and Alternative Medicine 2016*, 6495410.

Damery, S., Gratus, C., Grieve, R., Warmington, S., *et al.* (2011) 'The use of herbal medicines by people with cancer: A cross-sectional survey.' *British Journal of Cancer 104*(6), 927–933.

Dante, G., Bellei, G., Neri, I. and Facchinetti, F. (2014) 'Herbal therapies in pregnancy: What works?' *Current Opinions in Obstetrics and Gynecology 26*(2), 83–91.

Datta, S., Mahdi, F., Ali, Z., Jekabsons, M.B., *et al.* (2014) 'Toxins in botanical dietary supplements: Blue cohosh components disrupt cellular respiration and mitochondrial membrane potential.' *Journal of Natural Products 77*(1), 111–117.

Davis, E.L., Oh, B., Butow, P.N., Mullan, B.A. and Clarke, S. (2012) 'Cancer patient disclosure and patient–doctor communication of complementary and alternative medicine use: A systematic review.' *Oncologist 17*(11), 1475–1481.

Delmondao, M. (2016) 'Use of medicinal herbs during the childbearing year among direct-entry midwives in the Pacific Northwest.' Thesis. Available at www.google. com/search?q=use+of+herbs+in+midwifery%2C+USA&rlz=1C1CHBF_en-GBGB 781GB781&oq=use+of+herbs+in+midwifery%2C+USA&aqs=chrome.0.69i59.4310 j0j4&sourceid=chrome&ie=UTF-8

Dennehy, C., Tsourounis, C., Bui, L. and King, T.L. (2010) 'The use of herbs by California midwives.' *Journal of Obstetric, Gynecologic, & Neonatal Nursing 39*(6), 684–693.

Di Gaspero, N.C., Razlog, R., Patel, R. and Pellow, J. (2019) 'Perceived effectiveness of complementary medicine by mothers of infants with colic in Gauteng.' *Health SA 24*, 1175.

Di Minno, A., Frigerio, B., Spadarella, G., Ravani, S., *et al.* (2017) 'Old and new oral anticoagulants: Food, herbal medicines and drug interactions.' *Blood Reviews 31*(4), 193–203. Available at www.sciencedirect.com/science/article/pii/ S0268960X16300352?via%3Dihub

Dugoua, J.J., Perri, D., Seely, D., Mills, E. and Koren, G. (2008) 'Safety and efficacy of blue cohosh (*Caulophyllum thalictroides*) during pregnancy and lactation.' *The Canadian Journal of Clinical Pharmacology 15*(1), e66–e73.

Editorial (2018) 'Herbal assault: Liver toxicity of herbal and dietary supplements.' *The Lancet 3*, March. Available at www.thelancet.com/action/ showPdf?pii=S2468-1253%2818%2930011-6

Eid, A.M. and Jaradat, N. (2020) 'Public knowledge, attitude, and practice on herbal remedies used during pregnancy and lactation in West Bank Palestine.' *Frontiers in Pharmacology 11*(46). Available at https://pubmed.ncbi.nlm.nih.gov/32116721

Einion, A. (2016) 'Aromatherapy in midwifery practice.' *The Practising Midwife 19*(5), 12, 14–15.

Ekor, M. (2013) 'The growing use of herbal medicines: Issues relating to adverse reactions and challenges in monitoring safety.' *Frontiers in Pharmacology 4*, 177.

FDA (Food and Drug Administration) (2019) 'Drug products labeled as homeopathic; draft guidance for Food and Drug Administration staff and industry.' *Federal Register: The Daily Journal of the United States Government* 25 October. Available at www. federalregister.gov/documents/2019/10/25/2019-23335/drug-products-labeled-as-homeopathic-draft-guidance-for-food-and-drug-administration-staff-and

Fernandez, C. and Taylor, R. (2019) 'Homeopathic medicine will be banned by the NHS because it is a "misuse of public funds", after it emerges doctors prescribed alternative remedies 3,300 times last year.' *Daily Mail Online* 7 April. Available at www.dailymail.co.uk/health/article-6896733/Homeopathic-medicine-banned-NHS-misuse-public-funds.html

Finkel, R.S. and Zarlengo, K.M. (2004) 'Blue cohosh and perinatal stroke.' *The New England Journal of Medicine 351*(3), 302–303.

Frawley, J., Adams, J., Steel, A., Broom, A., Gallois, C. and Sibbritt, D. (2015) 'Women's use and self-prescription of herbal medicine during pregnancy: An examination of 1,835 pregnant women.' *Women's Health Issues 25*(4), 396–402.

Freeman, M., Ayers, C., Peterson, C. and Kansagara, D. (2019) 'Aromatherapy and essential oils: A map of the evidence.' *US Department of Veterans Affairs.* VA Evidence-Based Synthesis Program. Available at www.ncbi.nlm.nih.gov/books/NBK551017

Fukunaga, R., Morof, D., Blanton, C., Ruiz, A., Maro, G. and Serbanescu, F. (2020) 'Factors associated with local herb use during pregnancy and labor among women in Kigoma region, Tanzania, 2014–2016.' *BMC Pregnancy and Childbirth 20*(122). Available at https://bmcpregnancychildbirth.biomedcentral.com/articles/10.1186/s12884-020-2735-3

Gerdts, C., Raifman, S., Daskilewicz, K., Momberg, M., Roberts, S. and Harries, J. (2017) 'Women's experiences seeking informal sector abortion services in Cape Town, South Africa: A descriptive study.' *BMC Women's Health 17*(1), 95.

Ghazali, Y., Bello, I. and Kola-Mustapha, A. (2019) 'The use of herbal medicines amongst outpatients at the University of Ilorin Teaching Hospital (UITH), Ilorin, Kwara State – Nigeria.' *Complementary Therapies in Medicine 42*, 158–163.

Golec, M., Skórska, C., Mackiewicz, B., Gora, A. and Dutkiewicz, J. (2005) 'Respiratory effects of exposure to dust from herbs.' *Annals of Agricultural and Environmental Medicine 12*(1), 5–10.

Grand View Research (2019) *Aromatherapy Market Size Analysis Report by Product (Consumables, Equipment), by Mode of Delivery (Topical, Aerial, Direct Inhalation), by Application, by Distribution Channel, by End Use, and Segment Forecasts, 2019–2026.* Available at www.grandviewresearch.com/industry-analysis/aromatherapy-market

Green, R., Santoro, N., Allshouse, A.A., Neal-Perry, G. and Derby, C. (2017) 'Prevalence of complementary and alternative medicine and herbal remedy use in Hispanic and non-Hispanic white women: Results from the study of women's health across the nation.' *Journal of Alternative and Complementary Medicine 23*(10), 805–811.

Gunn, J.K., Rosales, C.B., Center, K.E., Nuñez, A., *et al.* (2016) 'Prenatal exposure to cannabis and maternal and child health outcomes: A systematic review and meta-analysis.' *BMJ Open 6*(4), e009986.

Guo, X. and Mei, N. (2016) 'Aloe vera: A review of toxicity and adverse clinical effects.' *Journal of Environmental Science and Health, Part C: Environmental Carcinogenesis Ecotoxicology Reviews 34*(2), 77–96.

Hall, H.G., Griffiths, D.L. and McKenna, L.G. (2011) 'The use of complementary and alternative medicine by pregnant women: A literature review.' *Midwifery 27*(6), 817–824.

Hall, H.G., Griffiths, D.L. and McKenna, L.G. (2013) 'Keeping childbearing safe: Midwives' influence on women's use of complementary and alternative medicine.' *International Journal of Nursing Practice 19*(4), 437–443.

Hall, H.G., McKenna, L.G. and Griffiths, D.L. (2012) 'Midwives' support for complementary and alternative medicine: A literature review.' *Women and Birth 25*(1), 4–12.

Hall, H.R. and Jolly, K. (2014) 'Women's use of complementary and alternative medicines during pregnancy: A cross-sectional study.' *Midwifery 30*(5), 499–505.

Hammer, K.A., Carson, C.A., Riley, T.V. and Nielsen, J.B. (2006) 'A review of the toxicity of *melaleuca alternifolia* (tea tree) oil.' *Food and Chemical Toxicology 44*(5), 616–625.

He, S.M., Chan, E. and Zhou, S.F. (2011) 'ADME properties of herbal medicines in humans: Evidence, challenges and strategies.' *Current Pharmaceutical Design 17*(4), 357–407.

Henson, J.B., Brown, C.L., Chow, S.C. and Muir, A.J. (2017) 'Complementary and alternative medicine use in United States adults with liver disease.' *Journal of Clinical Gastroenterology 51*(6), 564–570.

Hernandez, S., Oliveira, J.B. and Sharazian, T. (2017) 'How a training program is transforming the role of traditional birth attendants from cultural practitioners to unique health-care providers: A community case study in rural Guatemala.' *Frontiers in Public Health 5*, 11. Available at www.frontiersin.org/articles/10.3389/fpubh.2017.00111/full

Heydari, M., Heydari, H., Saadati, A., Gharehbeglou, M., Tafaroji, J. and Akbari, A. (2016) 'Ethnomedicine for neonatal jaundice: A cross-sectional survey in Qom, Iran.' *Journal of Ethnopharmacology 193*, 637–642.

Heywood, V.E. (2011) 'Ethnopharmacology, food production, nutrition and biodiversity conservation: Towards a sustainable future for indigenous peoples.' *Journal of Ethnopharmacology 137*, 1–15.

Hoang, M.L., Chen, C.H., Chen, P.C., Roberts, N.J., *et al.* (2016) 'Aristolochic acid in the etiology of renal cell carcinoma.' *Cancer Epidemiology, Biomarkers & Prevention 25*(12), 1600–1608.

Hsu, J. (2017) 'The hard truth about the rhino horn "aphrodisiac" market.' *Scientific American* 5 April. Available at www.scientificamerican.com/article/the-hard-truth-about-the-rhino-horn-aphrodisiac-market

Hua, M., Fan, J., Dong, H. and Sherer, R. (2017) 'Integrating traditional Chinese medicine into Chinese medical education reform: Issues and challenges.' *International Journal of Medical Education 8*, 126–127.

Hui, H., Tang, G. and Go, V.L.W. (2009) 'Hypoglycemic herbs and their action mechanisms.' *Chinese Medicine 4*, 11. Available at www.ncbi.nlm.nih.gov/pmc/articles/PMC2704217

Hull, T., Hilber, A.M., Chersich, M.F., Bagnol, B., *et al.* (2011) 'Prevalence, motivations, and adverse effects of vaginal practices in Africa and Asia: Findings from a multicountry household survey.' *Journal of Women's Health (Larchmt) 20*(7), 1097–1109.

Hunt, K. (2019) 'Chinese medicine gains WHO acceptance but it has many critics.' *CNN Health.* Available at https://edition.cnn.com/2019/05/24/health/traditional-chinese-medicine-who-controversy-intl/index.html

Illamola, S.M., Amaeze, O.U., Krepkova, L.V., Birnbaum, A.K., Karanam, A. *et al.* (2020) 'Use of Herbal Medicine by Pregnant Women: What Physicians Need to Know.' *Frontiers in pharmacology, 10*, 1483. Available at https://doi.org/10.3389/fphar.2019.01483

Iwata, N., Kainuma, M., Kobayashi, D., Kubota, T., *et al.* (2016) 'The relation between hepatotoxicity and the total coumarin intake from traditional Japanese medicines containing cinnamon bark.' *Frontiers in Pharmacology 7*, 174. Available at www.ncbi.nlm.nih.gov/pmc/articles/PMC4913087

Izzo, A.A., Hoon-Kim, S., Radhakrishnan, R. and Williamson, E.M. (2016) 'A critical approach to evaluating clinical efficacy, adverse events and drug interactions of herbal remedies.' *Phytotherapy Research 30*(5), 691–700.

Jalili, J., Askeroglu, U., Alleyne, B. and Guyuron, B. (2013) 'Herbal products that may contribute to hypertension.' *Plastic and Reconstructive Surgery 131*(1), 168–173.

Jambo, A., Mengistu, G., Sisay, M., Amare, F. and Edessa, D. (2018) 'Self-medication and contributing factors among pregnant women attending antenatal care at public hospitals of Harar town, Ethiopia.' *Frontiers in Pharmacology 9*, 1063.

James, P.B., Bah, A.J., Tommy, M.S., Wardle, J. and Steel, A. (2018) 'Herbal medicines use during pregnancy in Sierra Leone: An exploratory cross-sectional study.' *Women and Birth 31*(5), e302–e309.

James, P.B., Kaikai, A.I., Bah, A.J., Steel, A. and Wardle, J. (2019) 'Herbal medicine use during breastfeeding: A cross-sectional study among mothers visiting public health facilities in the Western area of Sierra Leone.' *BMC Complementary and Alternative Medicine 19*, 66.

John, L.J. and Shantakumari, N. (2015) 'Herbal medicines use during pregnancy: A review from the Middle East.' *Oman Medical Journal 30*(4), 229–236.

Johnson, C. (2014) 'Is homeopathy safe? A response to Posadzki et al.' *Journal of Alternative and Complementary Medicine 20*(1), 67–68.

Johnson, P.J., Kozhimannil, K.B., Jou, J., Ghildayal, M. and Rockwood, T.H. (2016) 'Complementary and Alternative Medicine (CAM) use among women of reproductive age in the United States.' *Women's Health Issues 26*(1), 40–47.

Johny, A.K., Cheah, W.L. and Razitasham, S. (2017) 'Disclosure of traditional and complementary medicine use and its associated factors to medical doctor in primary care clinics in Kuching Division, Sarawak, Malaysia.' *Evidence-Based Complementary and Alternative Medicine 2017*, 5146478.

Kaadaaga, H.F., Ajeani, J., Ononge, S., Alele, P.A., *et al.* (2014) 'Prevalence and factors associated with use of herbal medicine among women attending an infertility clinic in Uganda.' *BMC Complementary and Alternative Medicine 14*, 27. Available at https://doi.org/10.1186/1472-6882-14-27

Kam, P.C., Barnett, D.W. and Douglas, I.D. (2019) 'Herbal medicines and pregnancy: A narrative review and anaesthetic considerations.' *Anaesthesia and Intensive Care 24*, 310057X19845786.

Kandola, A. (2018) 'Kava kava: Benefits and safety concerns.' *Medical News Today* 17 December. Available at www.medicalnewstoday.com/articles/324015

Karsch-Völk, M., Barrett, B., Bauer, R., Ardjomand-Woelkart, K. and Linde, K. (2014) 'Echinacea for preventing and treating the common cold.' *Cochrane Database of Systematic Reviews 2014*, 2, CD000530.

Kawai, E., Takeda, R., Ota, A., Morita, E., *et al.* (2020) 'Increase in diastolic blood pressure induced by fragrance inhalation of grapefruit essential oil is positively correlated with muscle sympathetic nerve activity.' *The Journal of Physiological Sciences 70*(1), 2.

Kelak, J.A., Cheah, W.L. and Safii, R. (2018) 'Patient's decision to disclose the use of traditional and complementary medicine to medical doctor: A descriptive phenomenology study.' *Evidence-Based Complementary and Alternative Medicine 2018*, 4735234. Available at https://doi.org/10.1155/2018/4735234

Kennedy, D.A., Lupattelli, A., Koren, G. and Nordeng, H. (2013) 'Herbal medicine use in pregnancy: Results of a multinational study.' *BMC Complementary and Alternative Medicine 13*, 355.

Kennedy, D.A., Lupattelli, A., Koren, G. and Nordeng, H. (2016) 'Safety classification of herbal medicines used in pregnancy in a multinational study.' *BMC Complementary and Alternative Medicine 16*, 102.

Kıssal, A., Çevik Güner, Ü. and Batkın Ertürk, D. (2017) 'Use of herbal product among pregnant women in Turkey.' *Complementary Therapies in Medicine 30*, 54–60.

Koc, Z., Topatan, S. and Saglam, Z. (2012) 'Use of and attitudes toward complementary and alternative medicine among midwives in Turkey.' *European Journal of Obstetrics & Gynecology and Reproductive Biology 160*(2), 131–136.

Laelago, T., Yohannes, T. and Lemango, F. (2016) 'Prevalence of herbal medicine use and associated factors among pregnant women attending antenatal care at public health facilities in Hossana Town, Southern Ethiopia: Facility based cross sectional study.' *Archives of Public Health 74*, 7.

Lake, E.A. and Olana Fite, R. (2019) 'Low birth weight and its associated factors among newborns delivered at Wolaita Sodo University Teaching and Referral Hospital, Southern Ethiopia, 2018.' *International Journal of Pediatrics 2019*, 4628301.

Lee, A.H., Kabashneh, S., Tsouvalas, C.P., Rahim, U., *et al.* (2020) 'Proctocolitis from coffee enema.' *ACG Case Reports Journal 7*(1), e00292.

Li, L.Y., Cao, F.F., Su, Z.J., Zhang, Q.H., *et al.* (2015) 'Assessment of the embryotoxicity of four Chinese herbal extracts using the embryonic stem cell test.' *Molecular Medicine Reports 12*(2), 2348–2354.

Lin, C.Y., Chen, Y.J., Lee, S.H., Kuo, C.P., Lee, M.S. and Lee, M.C. (2019) 'Uses of dietary supplements and herbal medicines during pregnancy in women undergoing assisted reproductive technologies – A study of Taiwan birth cohort.' *Taiwanese Journal of Obstetrics & Gynecology 58*(1), 77–81.

Liu, Z., He, X., Wang, L., Zhang, Y., Hai, Y. and Gao, R. (2018) 'Chinese herbal medicine hepatotoxicity: The evaluation and recognition based on large-scale evidence database.' *Current Drug Metabolism 19*(14), 138–146.

Lombaerts, C. and Vanthuyne, H. (2018) 'Teaching midwives homeopathy – A Belgian pilot project.' *European Journal of Integrative Medicine 21*, August, 16–23.

MacPherson, R.D. and Kilminster, I. (2006) 'Neonatal epilepsy associated with maternal ingestion of blue cohosh.' *Journal of Pharmacy Practice and Research 36*, 4.

Manzalini, A. and Galeazzi, B. (2019) 'Explaining homeopathy with quantum electrodynamics.' *Homeopathy 108*(3), 169–176.

Maonga, A.R., Mahande, M.J., Damian, D.J. and Msuya, S.E. (2016) 'Factors affecting exclusive breastfeeding among women in Muheza District Tanga, Northeastern Tanzania: A mixed method community based study.' *Maternal and Child Health Journal 20*, 77–87.

Math, S.B., Moirangthem, S., Kumar, N.C. and Nirmala, M.C. (2015) 'Ethical and legal issues in cross-system practice in India: Past, present and future.' *The National Medical Journal of India 28*(6), 295–299.

Mathie, R.T., Ramparsad, N., Legg, L.A., Clausen, J., *et al.* (2017) 'Randomised, double-blind, placebo-controlled trials of non-individualised homeopathic treatment: Systematic review and meta-analysis.' *Systematic Reviews 6*(1), 63.

Matthews-King, A. (2019) 'World Health Organisation's recognition of traditional Chinese medicine "could push species into extinction".' *The Independent* 28 May. Available at www.independent.co.uk/news/health/china-medicine-wildlife-poaching-conservation-world-health-organisation-a8933061.html

Mayo Clinic (2017) 'St John's wort.' Available at www.mayoclinic.org/drugs-supplements-st-johns-wort/art-20362212

McIntyre, E., Foley, H., Diezel, H., Harnett, J., *et al.* (2020) 'Development and preliminarily validation of the Complementary Medicine Disclosure Index.' *Patient Education and Counseling 103*(6), 1237–1244. Available at www.sciencedirect.com/science/article/abs/pii/S0738399120300070

McLay, J.S., Pallivalappila, A.R., Shetty, A., Pande, B., Al Hail, M. and Stewart, D. (2016) '"Asking the right question": A comparison of two approaches to gathering data on "herbals" use in survey-based studies.' *PLoS One 11*(2), e0150140.

MHRA (Medicines and Healthcare products Regulatory Agency) (2014) 'Banned and restricted herbal ingredients.' Available at www.gov.uk/government/publications/list-of-banned-or-restricted-herbal-ingredients-for-medicinal-use/banned-and-restricted-herbal-ingredients

Mokgobi, M.G. (2014) 'Understanding traditional African healing.' *African Journal for Physical, Health Education, Recreation and Dance 20*(Suppl. 2), 24–34.

Mollart, L., Skinner, V., Adams, J. and Foureur, M. (2018) 'Midwives' personal use of complementary and alternative medicine (CAM) influences their recommendations to women experiencing a post-date pregnancy.' *Women and Birth 31*(1), 44–51.

Mollart, L., Stulz, V. and Foureur, M. (2019) 'Midwives' personal views and beliefs about complementary and alternative medicine (CAM): A national survey.' *Complementary Therapies in Clinical Practice 34*, 235–239.

Mothibe, M.E. and Sibanda, M. (2019) 'African Traditional Medicine: South African Perspective.' In C. Mordeniz (ed.) *Traditional and Complementary Medicine* (Chapter 3). Available at www.intechopen.com/books/traditional-and-complementary-medicine/african-traditional-medicine-south-african-perspective

Muhlack, S., Lemmer, W., Klotz, P., Müller, T., Lehmann, E. and Klieser, E. (2006) 'Anxiolytic effect of Rescue Remedy for psychiatric patients: A double-blind, placebo-controlled, randomized trial.' *Journal of Clinical Psychopharmacology 26*(5), 541–542.

Muñoz Balbontín, Y., Stewart, D., Shetty, A., Fitton, C.A. and McLay, J.S. (2019) 'Herbal medicinal product use during pregnancy and the postnatal period: A systematic review.' *Obstetrics & Gynecology 133*(5), 920–932.

Muñoz-Sellés, E., Vallès-Segalés, A. and Goberna-Tricas, J. (2013) 'Use of alternative and complementary therapies in labor and delivery care: A cross-sectional study of midwives' training in Catalan hospitals accredited as centers for normal birth.' *BMC Complementary and Alternative Medicine 13*, 318.

Münstedt, K., Maisch, M., Tinneberg, H.R. and Hübner, J. (2014) 'Complementary and alternative medicine (CAM) in obstetrics and gynaecology: A survey of office-based obstetricians and gynaecologists regarding attitudes towards CAM, its provision and cooperation with other CAM providers in the state of Hesse, Germany.' *Archives of Gynecology and Obstetrics 290*(6), 1133–1139.

Nalumansi, P.A., Kamatenesi-Mugisha, M. and Anywar, G. (2017) 'Medicinal plants used during antenatal care by pregnant women in Eastern Uganda.' *African Journal of Reproductive Health 21*(4), 33–44.

Nath, S.S., Pandey, C. and Roy, D. (2012) 'A near fatal case of high dose peppermint oil ingestion – Lessons learnt.' *Indian Journal of Anaesthesia 56*(6), 582–584.

Ng, J.Y. (2020) 'The regulation of complementary and alternative medicine professions in Ontario, Canada.' *Integrative Medicine Research 9*(1), 12–16.

Nguyen, J., Smith, L., Hunter, J. and Harnett, J.E. (2019) 'Conventional and complementary medicine health care practitioners' perspectives on interprofessional communication: A qualitative rapid review.' *Medicina (Kaunas) 55*(10), ii, E650.

Nicolussi, S., Drewe, J., Butterweck, V. and Meyer zu Schwabedissen, H.E. (2020) 'Clinical relevance of St. John's wort drug interactions revisited.' *British Journal of Pharmacology 177*(6), 1212–1226.

Nwaiwu, O. and Oyelade, O.B. (2016) 'Traditional herbal medicines used in neonates and infants less than six months old in Lagos Nigeria.' *Nigerian Journal of Paediatrics 43*(1), 40.

Nyeko, R., Tumwesigye, N.M. and Halage, A.A. (2016) 'Prevalence and factors associated with use of herbal medicines during pregnancy among women attending postnatal clinics in Gulu district, Northern Uganda.' *BMC Pregnancy and Childbirth 16*(1), 296.

Ohaja, M. and Murphy-Lawless, J. (2017) 'Unilateral collaboration: The practices and understandings of traditional birth attendants in southeastern Nigeria.' *Women and Birth 30*(4), e165–e171.

Ossei, P.P.S., Appiah-Kubi, A., Ankobea-Kokroe, F., Owusu-Asubonteng, G., *et al.* (2020) 'The culture of herbal preparations among pregnant women: A remedy or a suicide potion? A case report and mini review.' *Case Reports in Pathology 2020*, 6186147.

Palanisamy, A., Haller, C. and Olson, K.R. (2003) 'Photosensitivity reaction in a woman using an herbal supplement containing ginseng, goldenseal, and bee pollen.' *Journal of Toxicology: Clinical Toxicology 41*(6), 865–867.

Pallivalapila, A.R., Stewart, D., Shetty, A., Pande, B., Singh, R. and McLay, J.S. (2015) 'Use of complementary and alternative medicines during the third trimester.' *Obstetrics & Gynecology 125*(1), 204–211.

Panganai, T. and Shumba, P. (2016) 'The African Pitocin, a midwife's dilemma: The perception of women on the use of herbs in pregnancy and labour in Zimbabwe, Gweru.' *Pan African Medical Journal 25*, 9.

Pantano, F., Tittarelli, R., Mannocchi, G. and Zaami, S., *et al.* (2016) 'Hepatotoxicity induced by "the 3Ks": Kava, kratom and khat.' *International Journal of Molecular Sciences 17*(4), 580.

Peprah, P., Agyemang-Duah, W., Arthur-Holmes, F., Budu, H.I., *et al.* (2019) '"We are nothing without herbs": A story of herbal remedies use during pregnancy in rural Ghana.' *BMC Complementary and Alternative Medicine 19*(1), 65.

Pokladnikova, J., Meyboom, R.H.B., Meincke, R., Niedrig, D. and Russman, S. (2016) 'Allergy-like immediate reactions with herbal medicines: A retrospective study using data from VigiBase®.' *Drug Safety 39*(5), 455–464.

Posadzki, P., Watson, L.K., Alotaibi, A. and Ernst, E. (2013) 'Prevalence of use of complementary and alternative medicine (CAM) by patients/consumers in the UK: Systematic review of surveys.' *Clinical Medicine (London) 13*(2), 126–131.

Prasad, P., Tantia, O., Patle, N.M. and Mukherjee, J. (2012) 'Herbal enema: At the cost of colon.' *Journal of Minimal Access Surgery 8*(3), 104–106.

Rahmawati, R. and Bajorek, B.V. (2017) 'Self-medication among people living with hypertension: A review.' *Family Practice 34*(2), 147–153.

Ramesh, R. (2009) 'India moves to protect traditional medicines from foreign patents.' *The Guardian* 22 February. Available at www.theguardian.com/world/2009/feb/22/india-protect-traditional-medicines

Rashrash, M., Schommer, J.C. and Brown, L.M. (2017) 'Prevalence and predictors of herbal medicine use among adults in the United States.' *Journal of Patient Experience 4*(3), 108–113.

Rašković, A., Cvejić, J., Stilinović, N., Goločorbin-Kon, S., *et al.* (2014) 'Interaction between different extracts of *Hypericum perforatum L.* from Serbia and pentobarbital, diazepam and paracetamol.' *Molecules 19*(4), 3869–3882.

Razaghi, N., Aemmi, S.Z., Sadat Hoseini, A.S., Boskabadi, H., Mohebbi, T. and Ramezani, M. (2020) 'The effectiveness of familiar olfactory stimulation with lavender scent and glucose on the pain of blood sampling in term neonates: A randomized controlled clinical trial.' *Complementary Therapies in Medicine 49*, March, 102289.

Resende, M.M., Costa, F.E., Gardona, R.G., Araújo, R.G., Mundim, F.G. and Costa, M.J. (2014) 'Preventive use of Bach Flower Rescue Remedy in the control of risk factors for cardiovascular disease in rats.' *Complementary Therapies in Medicine 22*(4), 719–723.

Riang'a, R.M., Nangulu, A.K. and Broerse, J.E.W. (2018) 'Perceived causes of adverse pregnancy outcomes and remedies adopted by Kalenjin women in rural Kenya.' *BMC Pregnancy and Childbirth 18*(1), 408.

Rivas-Suárez, S.R., Águila-Vázquez, J., Suárez-Rodríguez, B., Vázquez-León, L., *et al.* (2017) 'Exploring the effectiveness of external use of Bach flower remedies on carpal tunnel syndrome: A pilot study.' *Journal of Evidence-Based Complementary and Alternative Medicine 22*(1), 18–24.

Royal Botanical Gardens, Kew (2017) *State of the World's Plants 2017*. Available at https://stateoftheworldsplants.org/2017/report/SOTWP_2017.pdf

Sabourian, R., Karimpour-Razkenari, E., Saeedi, M., Bagheri, M.S., *et al.* (2016) 'Medicinal plants used in Iranian traditional medicine (itm) as contraceptive agents.' *Current Pharmaceutical Biotechnology 17*(11), 974–985.

Sattari, M., Dilmaghanizadeh, M., Hamishehkar, H. and Mashayekhi, S.O. (2012) 'Self-reported use and attitudes regarding herbal medicine safety during pregnancy in Iran.' *Jundishapur Journal of Natural Pharmaceutical Products 7*(2), 45–49.

Scott, I. (2019) 'A "grave error": France to phase out coverage for homeopathy.' France 24. Available at www.france24.com/en/20190710-outrage-france-govt-cancels-coverage-homeopathic-medicine

Sensi, H., Buch, H., Ford, L. and Gama, R. (2019) 'Herbal remedies adulterated with glucocorticoids can cause Cushing's syndrome.' *BMJ Case Reports 12*(2), ii, bcr-2018-228443.

Shand, A.W., Walls, M., Chatterjee, R., Nassar, N. and Khambalia, A.Z. (2016) 'Dietary vitamin, mineral and herbal supplement use: A cross-sectional survey of before and during pregnancy use in Sydney, Australia.' *Australian and New Zealand Journal of Obstetrics and Gynaecology 56*(2), 154–161.

Shewamene, Z., Dune, T. and Smith, C.A. (2017) 'The use of traditional medicine in maternity care among African women in Africa and the diaspora: A systematic review.' *BMC Complementary and Alternative Medicine 17*, 382.

Shikov, A.N., Tsitsilin, A.N., Pozharitskaya, O.N., Makarov, V.G. and Heinrich, M. (2017) 'Traditional and current food use of wild plants listed in the Russian Pharmacopoeia.' *Frontiers in Pharmacology 21*(8), 841.

Sibbritt, D.W., Catling, C.J., Adams, J., Shaw, A.J. and Homer, C.S. (2014) 'The self-prescribed use of aromatherapy oils by pregnant women.' *Women and Birth 27*(1), 41–45.

Singh, A. and Zhao, K. (2017) 'Herb–drug interactions of commonly used Chinese medicinal herbs.' *International Review of Neurobiology 135*, 197–232.

Smeriglio, A., Tomaino, A. and Trombetta, D. (2014) 'Herbal products in pregnancy: Experimental studies and clinical reports.' *Phytotherapy Research 28*(8), 1107–1116.

Smith, T.J. and Ashar, B.H. (2019) 'Iron deficiency anemia due to high-dose turmeric.' *Cureus 11*(1), e3858.

Stanisiere, J., Mousset, P.-Y. and Lafay, S. (2018) 'How safe is ginger rhizome for decreasing nausea and vomiting in women during early pregnancy?' *Foods 7*(4), 50.

Stevens, J., Dahlen, H., Peters, K. and Jackson, D. (2011) 'Midwives' and doulas' perspectives of the role of the doula in Australia: A qualitative study.' *Midwifery 27*(4), 509–516.

Stewart, D., Pallivalappila, A.R., Shetty, A., Pande, B. and McLay, J.S. (2014) 'Healthcare professional views and experiences of complementary and alternative therapies in obstetric practice in North East Scotland: A prospective questionnaire survey.' *BJOG: An International Journal of Obstetrics & Gynaecology 121*(8), 1015–1019.

Stoddard, G.J., Archer, M., Shane-McWhorter, L., Bray, B.E., *et al.* (2015) 'Ginkgo and warfarin interaction in a large Veterans Administration population.' *AMIA Annual Symposium Proceedings 2015*, 1174–1183.

Strouss, L., Mackley, A., Guillen, U., Paul, D.A. and Locke, R. (2014) 'Complementary and alternative medicine use in women during pregnancy: Do their healthcare providers know?' *BMC Complementary and Alternative Medicine 14*, 85.

Stub, T., Quandt, S.A., Arcury, T.A., Sandberg, J.C., *et al.* (2016) 'Perception of risk and communication among conventional and complementary health care providers involving cancer patients' use of complementary therapies: A literature review.' *BMC Complementary and Alternative Medicine 8*(16), 353.

Swerts, S., van Gasse, A., Leysen, J., Faber, M., *et al.* (2014) 'Allergy to illicit drugs and narcotics.' *Clinical & Experimental Allergy 44*(3), 307–318.

Tabassum, N. and Ahmad, F. (2011) 'Role of natural herbs in the treatment of hypertension.' *Pharmacognosy Reviews 5*(9), 30–40.

Tariq, S., Wani, S., Rasool, W., Shafi, K., *et al.* (2019) 'A comprehensive review of the antibacterial, antifungal and antiviral potential of essential oils and their chemical constituents against drug-resistant microbial pathogens.' *Microbial Pathogenesis 134*, 103580.

Teschke, R. and Eickhoff, A. (2015) 'Herbal hepatotoxicity in traditional and modern medicine: Actual key issues and new encouraging steps.' *Frontiers in Pharmacology 6*, 72.

Tiran, D. (2012) 'Ginger to reduce nausea and vomiting during pregnancy: Evidence of effectiveness is not the same as proof of safety.' *Complementary Therapies in Clinical Practice 18*(1), 22–25.

Tiran, D. (2016) *Aromatherapy in Midwifery Practice*. London: Singing Dragon.

Tiran, D. (2018) *Complementary Therapies in Maternity Care: An Evidence-Based Approach*. London: Singing Dragon.

Tournier, A., Roberts, E.R. and Viksveen, P. (2013) 'Adverse effects of homeopathy: A systematic review of published case reports and case series – Comment by Tournier et al.' *International Journal of Clinical Practice 67*(4), 388–389.

Trabace, L., Tucci, P., Ciuffreda, L., Matteo, M., *et al.* (2015) '"Natural" relief of pregnancy-related symptoms and neonatal outcomes: Above all do no harm.' *Journal of Ethnopharmacology 174*, 396–402.

van der Helm, J.J., van der Loeff, M.F.S., de Vries, E., van der Veer, C., *et al.* (2019) 'Vaginal herb use and *Chlamydia trachomatis* infection: Cross-sectional study among women of various ethnic groups in Suriname.' *BMJ Open 9*(5), e025417.

Volqvartz, T., Vestergaard, A.L., Aagaard, S.K., Andreasen, M.F., *et al.* (2019) 'Use of alternative medicine, ginger and licorice among Danish pregnant women – A prospective cohort study.' *BMC Complementary and Alternative Medicine 19*(1), 5.

Walach, H., Lewith, G. and Jonas, W. (2013) 'Can you kill your enemy by giving homeopathy? Lack of rigour and lack of logic in the systematic review by Edzard Ernst and colleagues on adverse effects of homeopathy.' *The International Journal of Clinical Practice 67*(4), 385–386. Available at https://doi.org/10.1111/ijcp.12111

Walji, R., Boon, H., Barnes, J., Austin, Z., Baker, G.R. and Welsh, S. (2009) 'Adverse event reporting for herbal medicines: A result of market forces.' *Health Policy 4*(4), 77–90.

Wang, S., Zhang, C., Li, C., Li, D., *et al.* (2018) 'Efficacy of Chinese herbal medicine Zengru Gao to promote breastfeeding: A multicenter randomized controlled trial.' *BMC Complementary and Alternative Medicine 18*, 53.

Wei Yang, S., Koo, M. and Wang, Y.-H. (2015) 'The influence of Bach Rescue Remedy on the autonomic response to mental challenge in healthy Taiwanese women.' *Integrative Medicine Research 4*(1), 84, Supplement.

Welz, A.N., Emberger-Klein, A. and Menrad, K. (2018) 'Why people use herbal medicine: Insights from a focus-group study in Germany.' *BMC Complementary and Alternative Medicine 18*, 92.

WHO (World Health Organization) (2013) *WHO Traditional Medicine Strategy 2014–2023*. Geneva: WHO. Available at www.who.int/medicines/publications/traditional/trm_strategy14_23/en

WHO (2017) *Guidelines for Registration of Traditional Medicines in the WHO African Region*. Brazzaville and Geneva: Regional Office for Africa and Department of Essential Drugs and Medicines Policy. Available at www.afro.who.int/sites/default/files/2017-06/guide-reg-tm.pdf

WHO (2019) *WHO Global Report on Traditional and Complementary Medicine 2019.* Geneva: WHO. Available at www.who.int/traditional-complementary-integrative-medicine/WhoGlobalReportOnTraditionalAndComplementaryMedicine2019.pdf?ua=1%20)%202019

Wiebelitz, K.R., Goecke, T.W., Brach, J. and Beer, A.-M. (2013) 'Use of complementary and alternative medicine in obstetrics.' *British Journal of Midwifery 17,* 3. Available at https://doi.org/10.12968/bjom.2009.17.3.40079

Wolgast, E., Lindh-Åstrand, L. and Lilliecreutz, C. (2019) 'Women's perceptions of medication use during pregnancy and breastfeeding – A Swedish cross-sectional questionnaire study.' *Acta Obstetricia et Gynecologica Scandinavica 98*(7), 856–864.

Xinhua (2020) 'China approved 43 projects on TCM modernisation research.' Xinhuanet, 24 February. Available at www.xinhuanet.com/english/2020-02/24/c_138813952.htm

Yang, B., Xie, Y., Guo, M., Rosner, M.H., Yang, H. and Ronco, C. (2018) 'Nephrotoxicity and Chinese herbal medicine.' *Clinical Journal of the American Society of Nephrology 13*(10), 1605–1611.

Yuvaci, H.U., Yazici, E., Yazici, A.B. and Cevrioglu, S. (2019) 'How often do women use non-drug treatment methods for psychiatric symptoms during pregnancy and postpartum periods?' *Mental Illness 11*(1), 7988.

Zamawe, C., King, C., Jennings, H.M., Mandiwa, C. and Fottrell, E. (2018) 'Effectiveness and safety of herbal medicines for induction of labour: A systematic review and meta-analysis.' *BMJ Open 8*(10), e022499. doi:10.1136/bmjopen-2018-022499.

Zeni, A.L.B., Parisotto, A.V., Mattos, G. and de Santa Helena, E.T. (2017) 'Use of medicinal plants as home remedies in Primary Health Care in Blumenau – State of Santa Catarina, Brazil.' *Ciência & Saúde 22*(8), 2703. Available at www.scielo.br/pdf/csc/v22n8/1413-8123-csc-22-08-2703.pdf [article in Portuguese].

Zheng, T., Yao, D., Chen, W., Hu, H., Oi Lam Ung, C. and Harnett, J. (2019) 'Healthcare providers' role regarding the safe and appropriate use of herbal products by breastfeeding mothers: A systematic literature review.' *Complementary Therapies in Clinical Practice 35,* 131–147.

Subject Index

Note: Topics with major mentions, substantial information or given particular emphasis are indicated by page numbers in **bold**.

Author Index

About the Author

Denise Tiran, HonDUniv, FRCM, MSc, PGCEA, is an internationally renowned authority on maternity complementary medicine, having pioneered the subject as a midwifery specialism since the early 1980s. She is Chief Executive Officer and Education Director for Expectancy, an independent education company providing complementary therapies courses for midwives, doulas and therapists. Denise was awarded an Honorary Doctorate by the University of Greenwich in October 2020 and a Fellowship of the Royal College of Midwives in 2018 in recognition of her work in this field.